Lose Your FINAL 15

Lose Your
FINAL
15

Dr. Ro's Plan to Lose Your Last 15 Pounds by Eating 15 Servings a Day

ROVENIA M. BROCK, PhD

RODALE.

This book is intended as a reference volume only, not as a medical manual. The information given
here is designed to help you make informed decisions about your health. It is not intended as a
substitute for any treatment that may have been prescribed by your doctor. If you suspect that you
have a medical problem, we urge you to seek competent medical help.

The information in this book is meant to supplement, not replace, proper exercise training.
All forms of exercise pose some inherent risks. The editors and publisher advise readers
to take full responsibility for their safety and know their limits. Before practicing the exercises
in this book, be sure that your equipment is well-maintained, and do not take risks
beyond your level of experience, aptitude, training, and fitness. The exercise and dietary programs
in this book are not intended as a substitute for any exercise routine or dietary regimen
that may have been prescribed by your doctor. As with all exercise and dietary programs,
you should get your doctor's approval before beginning.

Mention of specific companies, organizations, or authorities in this book does not imply
endorsement by the author or publisher, nor does mention of specific companies, organizations,
or authorities imply that they endorse this book, its author, or the publisher.

Internet addresses and telephone numbers given in this book were accurate
at the time it went to press.

© 2016 by Rovenia M. Brock, PhD

All rights reserved. No part of this publication may be reproduced or transmitted in any form or by
any means, electronic or mechanical, including photocopying, recording, or any other information
storage and retrieval system, without the written permission of the publisher.

Rodale books may be purchased for business or promotional use or for special sales.
For information, please write to:
Special Markets Department, Rodale Inc., 733 Third Avenue, New York, NY 10017

Printed in the United States of America

Rodale Inc. makes every effort to use acid-free ♾, recycled paper ♻.

Before and after photos courtesy of Dr. Riggins, MASC

Book design by Christina Gaugler

Library of Congress Cataloging-in-Publication Data is on file with the publisher.

ISBN 978–1–62336–801–2

Distributed to the trade by Macmillan

2 4 6 8 10 9 7 5 3 1 hardcover

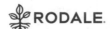

For Larvenia L. Brock and Rosetta Hyman Lewis, who taught me by example that love is the single most emotion to sustain humankind. For my husband, Murray, who has loved me with an open heart unconditionally, without fail for 15 years.

For Della Bannister, a legend among nutrition professionals who modeled excellence professionally and personally and who saw in me a yearning to use what she taught me to be of service to others. You have a permanent place in my heart. RIP.

For Simba, my companion and our family in cocker spaniel form, a warrior who sees the good in all and who never gives up, even when others doubt what you're made of. You inspire me.

For the scores of you who struggle with weight issues and who search for solutions, may you know kindness in the face of judgment, love in the face of disdain, and progress over perfection always. It is my sincere hope that this work helps you to get closer to the life you envision. Together we can do this!

CONTENTS

INTRODUCTION

Although I didn't realize it at the time, I started writing this book when I was 9 years old. My mother, Larvenia Brock, had been diagnosed with stomach cancer the year I was born. She had fought it off for years, but by the time I was 9, she was dying. She made many visits to a hospital in Washington, DC, that year, and I often went with her. While she met with her doctors, I spent time with her friend Ruby Cavanaugh, one of the hospital's dietitians.

Mrs. Cavanaugh taught patients how to improve their health by changing their diets. She educated people with ailments such as heart disease, diabetes, kidney disease, and cancer about how their dietary choices could help them—or hurt them.

As a child, I had only a vague understanding of Mrs. Cavanaugh's work with sick patients. And I certainly didn't comprehend the complex relationship between diet and health. But looking back, I realize that during those visits with Mrs. Cavanaugh, I began connecting some very important dots. And I started to hear the faint whisper of my life's calling.

My family ate a traditional Southern diet. We feasted regularly on deep-fried chicken, pork chops smothered in rich gravy, country ham, fried salt fish, hoecake, scrapple, chitlins, greens seasoned with fatback, potato salad smothered in mayonnaise, and a cornucopia of other dishes laden with fat, salt, and sugar. These foods brought us together; made from recipes passed down for generations, they represented our Southern culture and our family heritage.

Just as these Southern dishes were a part of the fabric of my childhood, so too was the presence of disease and disability. My grandparents, uncles, and aunts experienced a long list of health problems, including diabetes, hypertension, stroke, glaucoma, various kinds of cancer, and peripheral vascular disease, which my family called "poor circulation." Many of my relatives, neighbors, and family friends were overweight or obese.

Looking back, it should have come as no surprise to me on the playground the day that a friend announced, "My daddy had to have his legs cut off because of dia-bee-tees." Eventually, three of my maternal uncles would require limb amputations because of complications from peripheral vascular disease. At the age of 9, I started to understand, in a rudimentary way, that my community's eating habits were killing them. That connection stayed with me during adolescence, and when it came time for me to decide what to study in college at Virginia State University, I chose nutrition.

In college, I learned the many ways in which food influences our health. I realized that my mother's diet and weight almost certainly contributed to her stomach cancer and her early death. I discovered why my uncles lost limbs to diabetes and peripheral vascular disease. And, with a very heavy heart, I came to understand how much suffering and death in my family and my community could have been postponed or prevented if someone had taught the people I loved how to eat a healthier diet.

Without hesitation, I embraced the role of nutrition educator. I followed in Mrs. Cavanaugh's footsteps, working in hospitals and nursing homes educating patients with heart disease and diabetes on ways to improve their health by managing their diets. At the University of Maryland Medical System in Baltimore, I taught patients how to live and thrive after having coronary artery bypass surgery. Later I worked in the renal and critical care units at Howard University Hospital—ironically, the same hospital where I had sat with Mrs. Cavanaugh all those years earlier—using my nutrition skills and knowledge to improve the quality of patients' lives.

Working with patients was hugely satisfying for me. So many of my patients reminded me of my family and the wonderful, warm people in the LeDroit Park community in which I'd grown up. I felt that by helping them I was honoring my mother and all of the other people I loved whose health had been destroyed by poor diets and excess weight. But I wanted to do more. I wanted to be able to help more people than just the patients who came through my hospital. I realized that the best way to reach large numbers of people about the connections between diet and health was to take to the airways. So I went back to school and earned a master's degree in community nutrition and broadcast journalism and then a doctoral degree in nutritional sciences from Howard University.

Since then, I've made it my mission to reach out to as many people as possible through the media. I have hosted local and national radio and television shows. I've written extensively about nutrition and weight loss and the impact of both on health and quality of life. I've also written about how to break bad health habits, especially those considered to sabotage lasting weight-loss success. On *The Dr. Oz Show*, I created a program that guided over a half-million Americans to lose more than 5 million collective pounds.

Through my 28 years as a practicing nutritionist, it has become crystal clear to me that diet and exercise are the foundation of a healthy lifestyle. About 80 percent of the weight-loss process is due to diet, but 20 percent has everything to do with physical activity. The two go hand in hand. For my entire career, I've made it my mission to learn everything there is to know about healthy living so I could pass it on to you and to all of the other people who need help making choices about diet and fitness.

Although I have a PhD in nutrition, not all of my knowledge comes from textbooks. Despite everything I know about food, exercise, and health, the truth is that I've had my own struggles with diet and weight. Up until my midtwenties, I was quite thin, weighing in at about 100 pounds. But like a lot of black women, I worried that men wouldn't find me attractive unless I put a little more meat on my bones. This is a message that many women of color continue to hear now; I believe it is one of the reasons that obesity is a bigger problem in the African American and Latino communities than it is among other races. I can't believe it when I look back at those years, but I won't lie to you: I actually started overeating on a regular basis in order to appear more desirable to men. Gobbling up steak and cheese subs, ice cream, and an embarrassing array of junk food, I piled on 30 pounds. Friends and relatives congratulated me on my curves.

Eventually, when I was in my thirties, I took a look at myself and realized how foolish I'd been to gain all that extra weight. During the years that followed, I lost it and gained it back a few times, yo-yoing back and forth until I finally figured out how to follow my own advice and keep the weight off for good through diet and exercise.

All of this has led me to where I am right now. The book in your hands is the culmination of my decades of experience as a nutrition educator, a woman who has struggled with her own weight, and the child of a family and a community that has suffered the devastating effects of poor diet and excess weight.

This book, which can trace its history back to the broken heart of a 9-year-old girl in Washington, DC, brings together the knowledge, advice, and inspiration that made it possible for me to help thousands and thousands of people (and myself) lose weight and regain health by making life-saving diet changes. This is the book that I wish my mother could have read before being taken from me; or that my uncles could have read before having their limbs amputated; or that my beautiful guardian Rosetta Lewis, who raised me, could have read before experiencing heart disease, high blood pressure, and breast cancer. It is a book that I want you—and every other one of God's children—to read and use so that you can start making choices that will give you a long, healthy, happy life.

In the pages that follow, you will see that I have developed a program composed of three phases, 15 days each, on which you will eat 15 servings of delicious, nutritious, metabolism-boosting foods daily to help you lose weight. The first phase is probably the most difficult, but trust me, it is the most effective and quickest way to see the results of getting to your goal weight. And it may sound like it would be hard to do, but don't balk at the idea of eating 15 servings of food a day, because it's easier than you think. It is doable, simple, and sensible. I'm not asking you to eat 15 *times* a day, but rather to eat the correct portions of foods you're used to eating every day. What's different is that I have developed a plan with built-in macronutrients and calories ranging from 1,200 to 1,400 that you don't have to count. So the amount of servings you'll be eating will help you to shed unwanted pounds. What's more, after eating this way, you will be equipped with the tools needed to eat anywhere, whether it's at home or away. And you will gain the necessary knowledge to eyeball correct food portions, which prevents overeating and helps you to stick to your prescribed calorie budget.

ABOUT THE BOOK

Weight loss, diet change, and fitness can be overwhelming. This is especially true if you're facing a mountain-size goal—if you've got a lot of pounds to lose, or your diet is nothing but junk food, or you haven't exercised in a very long time (or ever). I get it. This stuff is hard. If it were easy, you wouldn't need a book like this.

But here's the thing: If you break one big goal into lots of smaller goals, you're much more likely to succeed and far less likely to feel overwhelmed. That's the philosophy behind my Final 15 (F-15) Plan. Based on the work I've done with thousands of patients, I've discovered that breaking everything up into units of 15 makes insurmountable challenges much easier to accomplish. I call this "The Rule of 15," and it's the backbone of all of the recommendations that I make in this book.

The F-15 Plan is an easy-to-follow diet and exercise plan that works with your body type, whether you tend to gain weight all over your body, just in the belly area, or on the hips and thighs or, dare I say—gulp—booty. For each body type, I provide a different strategy to help you lose all of your excess weight, including your Final 15 pounds.

Less Body Fat, More Energy

Using the F-15 Plan, you'll permanently lose belly fat, a problem that women and men alike confront day after day. You'll feel energized because the plan helps you choose foods that are best for *your* body. You'll also learn to detect and avoid food sensitivities that may be causing you to hold on to excess weight and that zap your energy, as well.

The F-15 Plan is simple and will fit any lifestyle; whether you're a student or a truck driver, an office worker or a store clerk, a deskbound engineer or an always-on-your-feet choir director, a teacher or a firefighter, or anything else in-between—this is the plan for you.

How can a healthy eating plan fit such a wide range of needs for such a diverse audience? By taking into account the need we all have for peak performance and energy. We are busy! We have families to raise, jobs to do, responsibilities to shoulder. So we all need an eating and exercise plan that can fit into the never-ending demands in our lives. I kept all that in mind when I created the F-15 Plan. To help you in your quest to be the best you, I have developed a diet that will not only help you lose weight but also help you breeze through plateaus and keep it off, all 15 pounds at a time.

The F-15 Plan is about permanent weight loss. There are no tricks or gimmicks, just a realistic plan that you can use to lose weight, lower your risk of disease, and live with for the rest of your life.

Here's how it works.

AN EASY, SENSIBLE FOOD PLAN

The F-15 Eating Plan consists of three 15-day phases. In each phase, you get to enjoy 15 servings of food per day. Tracking servings—rather than calories, fat grams, exchanges, or other units—is an easy, realistic way to eat the right amount of food for successful weight loss. And when you move to maintenance mode, you'll be glad that you kept track of realistic food servings and portions that you can use everywhere you go, both at home and away.

In Phase 1, you will eat power-packed foods, including vegetables and lean proteins. This helps you to kick-start weight loss and get your body to a clean and lean state.

In Phase 2, you will eat often and early so you can rev up your metabolism and prevent overeating. Foods in this phase include the same tasty, high-protein choices found in Phase 1, including eggs, low-fat dairy, vegetables, beans, seeds, and legumes, with the addition of fruit.

In Phase 3, you will be able to add in sprouted high-protein whole grains. This phase focuses on eating a variety of whole foods to keep yourself full for longer periods of time without overeating.

In each phase, you'll learn to identify the best foods for your lifestyle and body type as well as the triggers that derail your progress. And you'll eat tasty, easy-to-prepare foods that give you more energy, shrink belly fat, and improve your overall health and longevity.

QUICK, SIMPLE, AND DELICIOUS RECIPES

In the F-15 Plan, I've included tasty, delicious recipes for each phase—which gives you everything you need to be successful. Most of these recipes can be prepared in 15 minutes or less! These easy-to-make recipes will fit perfectly into your meal plan and your busy schedule. I know how important that is. I've coached clients for nearly three decades, and I'm no fool; I understand that you live in a time-starved world and that you have to make the most of your limited time while continuing to run here and there as you parent, answer to the demands of your job, and try to look and feel your best at the same time. It's a daunting process, but with the F-15 Plan, you can beat the defeat you may have experienced in the past and lose weight for good this time.

FABULOUS NO-FAIL FITNESS ROUTINES

The recommended goal for exercise is at least 30 minutes a day, most days of the week—and more if you really want to rev up exercise. But if you aren't already in an exercise habit, the thought of working out 30-plus minutes daily can be hugely overwhelming. That's why, as with everything else in my F-15 Plan, we'll start with 15-minute workout chunks. This allows you to start with one exercise unit per day, establish an exercise habit, and then go up from there.

My no-fail exercise plan includes belly-banishing, strength-training exercises that feel less like work and more like a fresh, new way of life, even for those of you whose only exercise has been running late and jumping to conclusions.

STEADY, PERMANENT WEIGHT LOSS

My clients find that losing weight 15 pounds at a time is doable and lasting, regardless of the number of pounds they have to lose. If you have, say, 45 pounds to lose, it's much easier to think of losing 15 pounds three times than to worry about losing an entire 45 pounds at once. You'll start by focusing on that first 15. Then, once you meet that goal, you can think about the next 15.

Science has shown us that people enjoy greater success by tackling their weight-loss problems in small increments. Most of my clients find that losing weight this way gets them consistent, lasting results. It works for them regardless of the number of pounds they have to lose, whether it's 15 pounds or 115. What's more, they are far more likely to stay the course when they see results.

The good news is that losing just 15 pounds can have an amazing impact on your health no matter what size you are. Research shows that overweight or obese people who lose as little as 5 to 10 percent of their weight start seeing dramatic reductions in medical risks. For example, diabetes risk drops significantly with a loss of just 5 to 10 percent of your body weight. For someone who weighs 200 pounds, that's a weight loss of 10 to 20 pounds—which really is a very attainable goal. Losing that first 15 pounds may not get you back into the jeans you wore in high school, but it can lower your risk of heart disease and diabetes, improve your blood sugar, increase your sensitivity to insulin, lower your blood pressure, and decrease inflammation. Furthermore, once you lose the first 15 pounds, you've proven to yourself that you have the power to do it over again and again, if you need to.

IMPORTANT NEW EATING BEHAVIORS

Success isn't just about eating the right foods. It's about changing the way you think about food. That's why the F-15 Plan focuses on changing your eating habits as well as the foods you choose. I'll show you how to redirect emotional eating and how to pinpoint the factors that push you off course. And I'll help you discover how to curb cravings and halt stress-eating for good.

You'll also master the art (yes, it's an artful process) of avoiding late-night snacking, one of the biggest roadblocks to weight-loss success. And you will be empowered to forge ahead, without self-doubt and deprecation. As your coach, I will hold your hand and have your back to get you through the entire process.

INSPIRATION THAT GOES DEEP

Losing weight requires motivation and inspiration. Most people who lose weight and keep it off do so not simply because they have a surplus of willpower but because they are motivated to do so. They win at the weight-loss game because motivation and encouragement work, especially when willpower is in short supply. Using techniques that work for my clients, I will share motivational and inspirational tools and tips throughout the book to help you stick to the process during moments of weakness. As you work toward becoming self-motivated, I want you to remember that I'll be with you, guiding you every step of the way, throughout your weight-loss program.

The Whole **F-15** Package

Imagine enjoying 15 servings a day of the tastiest, easiest-to-prepare, most power-packed foods you will ever eat.

Visualize yourself exercising in 15-minute chunks, doing muscle-building moves that give you energy, build strength, and rev up your metabolism.

Envision taking 15 minutes of your day to nourish and refresh your mind and to feed your soul, letting go of the stresses of the day.

That, in a nutshell, is the F-15 Plan.

Sure, you may have tried to lose weight before. But you threw in the towel, because the foods didn't suit you, or you pushed yourself to do too much exercise, or you were so focused on achieving weight loss that you forgot to give yourself time to relax and restore. That won't happen with the F-15 Plan because it is tailored to your specific needs, lifestyle, likes, and dislikes. What's not to like about that? Plus, the F-15 Plan is easy, because I've done most of the work for you. Not only does it include meal plans and recipes, but I've given you shopping lists, as well.

I encourage you to read on to find real foods and easy-to-do moves that you can incorporate into your daily life as it is now. That's right. I'm not asking you to become someone else in order to reach your goal. You are already the superstar of your own life, so why not live it to the fullest, in your best body? You can and will do this, because the individualized meal plan (made just for you, not the entire universe—as if that would work) will be tailored to your needs with the foods you enjoy. You don't even have to give up dessert!

Remember: I helped more than a half-million Americans lose over 5 million pounds with the F-15 Plan on *The Dr. Oz Show*. I can help you, too.

Now all I need is your buy-in and willingness to love yourself enough to give YOU a try for a really great outcome. So say it with me: "I *can* do this!" Louder, like you're for real! Say it! "I *can* do this!" Now take a deep breath. Turn the page, and let's get started!

Part I

GETTING STARTED

Chapter 1

WHAT IS THE F-15 PHILOSOPHY?

Nothing tastes as good as weight loss feels.
—Dr. Ro

Okay. Raise your hand if you feel like a failure.

Your hand went up, didn't it? I know it did. And if it didn't, it's probably because you're not being completely honest with yourself.

How do I know you feel like a failure? Because that's how just about everyone who picks up a weight-loss book feels. I can read you like a book, honey. You have extra pounds to lose—maybe just a few, maybe a lot more than that. You've lost weight before—maybe a few times, maybe a lot of times. But it always comes back; you always regain the pounds you lost, plus a few more. You feel frustrated, angry, and annoyed with yourself that you can't lose weight for good. You feel like a failure, right?

Listen, I get it. I yo-yoed back and forth with a few extra dress sizes myself. I was skinny as a stick into my twenties, but then I got it into my head that I needed some curves to catch men's eyes. This is something a lot of women of color are used to hearing even today, when we should all know better. "Get some meat on your bones," my family told me. "You look like a little girl, not a woman!" So when I was in my mid twenties, even though I was a nutritionist practicing in hospitals and nursing homes with a head full of knowledge about what a healthy diet should be, I began what I now think of as the "fool's diet." Yes, I actually began intentionally overeating and basically doing the opposite of what I knew was best for my health—eating giant portions, filling up before bedtime, having big desserts. In no time at all, I got the curves I was looking for— about 30 pounds worth in all.

Friends and family congratulated me left and right. But after a couple years, I realized I just didn't like the way all that weight felt and looked on me. So I decided to lose the extra pounds that I was dragging around. I stopped shoveling food onto my plate, stopped eating steak and cheese subs big enough for three people, and started following more of the dietary advice I was delivering to my patients at work every day. I also started working out zealously with a personal trainer. Before I knew it, the weight came off. Success! Hey, that wasn't so hard.

Up and Down

Unfortunately, the story doesn't end there. As my zeal for exercise fizzled, my weight ballooned back up. I gained those pounds back. Then I lost them again. And I gained them back again. You know how this story goes, I'm sure. This is your story, too. It's a story that plays out again and again, and the plotline is always the same. We lose weight and we feel good. Then we gain it back and feel bad. And throughout it all, we feel like failures, because we can't keep that darn weight off. Our closets are sectioned off into thin clothes, medium clothes, and fat clothes. I bounced back and forth from one dress size to another and still another so many times I could have opened a clothing store for women of at least three different sizes.

Finally, thank God, I figured things out and lost the weight for good. Yes, you guessed it: I lost that Final 15 and kept it off for good. How did I do it? Not by starving myself or following ridiculous fad diets that eliminate entire food groups. Nor did I do it by pledging my soul to an extreme fitness program that required hours and hours in the gym each week. Like you, I wanted a final solution. I wanted to lose weight for the last time and not gain it back. I was tired of feeling like a constant failure.

And I'm sure you are, too. That's why I created the F-15 Plan. It's designed to help you get back to a weight at which you feel your best, most comfortable, and happiest. Not only will my plan help change how your body looks, but it will also alter the way you feel about yourself. Together, we'll banish the word *failure* from your vocabulary. I will help you lose all the weight you need to lose and keep it off for good.

Why 15?

I call my plan the Final 15 because I know how overwhelming weight loss and diet change can be. No matter how much weight you have to lose—whether it's 10 pounds or 100—you're far more likely to succeed if you don't feel overwhelmed by your goal. I'm not saying you shouldn't try to lose a lot of weight. If you're 50, 75, or even 100 pounds overweight, I am totally with you on your desire to drop those extra pounds. But you don't have to do it all at once. As the old saying goes, a journey of a thousand miles starts with a single step. And losing a big amount of weight starts with a really reasonable goal: losing 15 pounds.

As the old saying goes, a journey of a thousand miles starts with a single step. And losing a big amount of weight starts with a really reasonable goal: losing 15 pounds.

With the F-15 Plan, I'll help you lose the first 15 pounds, the final 15 pounds, and any number of pounds in the middle. And I'll show you how to keep that last 15 pounds off for good, so you'll never have to lose it again. Wouldn't that be a blessing?

I also make weight loss easier by breaking down my diet plan into 15-day phases. I don't ask you to count calories, carbs, fat grams, or any of that other nonsense; instead, keeping it simple, I recommend 15 daily servings of right-size portions of healthy foods. And I make it easier to create a worthwhile exercise habit by giving you 15-minute workouts.

When it comes to weight loss, I've learned another really important lesson: The easier the plan is to follow, the more likely you are to succeed. That's why I've designed the F-15 Plan with simplicity in mind. I know how busy you are and what your life looks like. You're a parent helping your kids with homework and driving them all over town for sports, play dates, and educational enrichment. You're a business owner with deadlines to meet and staff to supervise. You're a student working hard to get an A in every class while working nights and weekends to pay tuition bills. You're an office worker whose nine-to-five work spills over into nights and weekends. You're a shift-worker trying to juggle your job and the needs of your family. You're a teacher, a nurse, a daycare provider, a store clerk. Maybe you're single, looking for that perfect partner, or maybe you've been married for decades. No matter what you do, who you are, or which responsibilities keep you awake at night, I get it—you're busy, you're stressed, you're constantly on the run, and you don't have the time to devote hours a day to your weight-loss plan.

That's why simplicity is the name of the game in the F-15 Plan. It takes the realities of your life into account, providing an easy-to-follow plan that will fit beautifully into your life.

What You're Up Against

Believe me. I get it. You've worked out, cut calories, and deprived yourself, all in hopes of getting rid of the stubborn pounds that have plagued you. Maybe you wanted to drop the baby weight but the belly bulge still lingers. Or maybe you're a hot guy (I see you) and you know it, but the extra weight you've worked so hard to drop won't, well, budge. Stubborn! I know. I feel your pain. You are not alone.

Two-thirds of American adults are overweight or obese. And one-third of American children are overweight or obese. Let's face it, the fact that in at least 12 states in the United States 30 percent of the population is considered obese speaks volumes about the epidemic we face as a country. But don't let these numbers scare you. I've worked with thousands of people who have managed to lose weight and keep it off. It's not as hard as you think; all you need are strategies that work, along with a commitment to do what it takes. I have the strategies, you have the desire—together we can beat the numbers!

An Abundance of Energy

In addition to fitting into your busy life, the F-15 Plan does something else amazing. It actually increases your energy levels so that you'll be better able to handle your life challenges. My clients are amazed at how energetic they feel when they start following the F-15 Plan. Within days, they feel less tired, less stressed, more invigorated, and more excited about life. This happens for several reasons.

Energy-boosting foods. The F-15 Plan includes an array of foods that infuse you with energy. Packed with vitamins, minerals, antioxidants, and other energy-fueling nutrients, F-15 foods give your body everything it needs to function at its best.

Energy-boosting fitness routines. We all need exercise, but too much activity—or the wrong kind of fitness routines—can wear you out. Instead, a smart exercise strategy like the one in the F-15 Plan can get you off the couch, build up your fitness level gradually, and give you energy while burning calories and building muscle. I don't ask you to do too much too soon; I've seen plenty of people ramp up their exercise commitment too fast, only to give it up within days because they feel exhausted and sore. Stick with me and you'll get all the benefits of fitness—including daily bursts of energy—without the downsides that over-the-top fitness fads can have.

Energy-boosting lifestyle choices. One of the things I'm going to talk to you about in this book is getting enough sleep—7 to 8 hours a night for most people. Adequate sleep is crucial for weight loss because it allows appetite-related hormones to do their jobs and help with weight loss rather than hinder it. And sleep gives you extra energy! When you get enough sleep and feel well rested, you have the energy you need to make smart choices throughout your day. Plus, having more energy makes it possible to have an active and fulfilling love life.

Energy-boosting thought strategies. Having the right mindset helps tremendously with weight loss. If you're not sure whether or not you believe that, look back at the last time you felt angry, irritated, or annoyed and think about what kinds of foods you chose to put in your mouth while you were experiencing those feelings. Lots of fat, sugar, and salt, am I right? I'm not promising to make your life a bed of roses or to take away all of the stresses that cause difficult emotions. But I will give you this: thought strategies that can energize your mind and help you to restructure food-related thinking patterns that cause you stress and contribute to poor choices. It's amazing: Practicing a few simple relaxation strategies can help you feel more energetic throughout the day and help you focus on making choices that support rather than detract from your goals.

Once you get into the swing of the F-15 Plan, you'll start feeling better than you have in a long time—perhaps in years. Combine this with the happiness you'll feel when the pounds start to come off, and believe me, life will be great!

Size Matters

Now that you understand what I had in mind when I designed the F-15 Plan, let's talk about size—serving size, that is. There are two main problems with the standard American diet: what we eat, and how much we eat. We'll talk about what's included in the F-15 Plan later, but first let's spend a little time on how much we eat.

Over the past few decades, average portion sizes in the United States have grown significantly. This is especially true in restaurants, where portion sizes have doubled or tripled in the past 20 years. When restaurants supersize their meals, it doesn't just make us eat too much when we're out to lunch or dinner. It actually changes the way we think about portion sizes, setting up a new "normal" in our brains. With these mammoth portions in mind, we serve ourselves extra at home, too.

Everything is bigger these days. Bagels have doubled in size. Cheeseburgers come with two or even three thick patties instead of one thin one. Fries are served in shovel-size containers, and soda cups are as big as buckets. "Single-serving" bags of potato chips are nearly three times bigger than they used to be. According to one analysis, this portion distortion can contribute as much as 500,000 extra calories to your diet in just 1 year. No wonder so many Americans are overweight!

Even when we choose the healthiest foods, our serving sizes can be too big. Healthy snacks such as guacamole, hummus, and nuts contain lots of fantastic, healthful nutrients, but if you aren't careful, you can eat too much. What looks like a single serving of nuts to the untrained eye, for example, could contain 300 or 400 calories, giving a snack as many calories as—or more calories than—a meal.

For all of these reasons, one of the most important parts of the F-15 Plan is to focus on serving sizes. I'll show you what serving sizes for various foods should be. If you're accustomed to oversize meals, these portions may seem a little small. But the truth is, they're the serving sizes that we all should be eating.

To make it easier for you, I'll also provide visual guides to estimate portion sizes. When a serving size is simple—a medium apple, for example—it's easy to grab a single serving without thinking too much about it. But with things like nuts, meat, and other foods, having a visual guide can help. If you like to measure and weigh, that's fine. But remember, I want things to be easy for you, and if you have to look around for measuring spoons, measuring cups, or a kitchen scale every time you're having something to eat, I consider that a roadblock that should be removed.

F-15 Self-Assessment Test: Where Are You Now?

In the pages that follow, you'll learn many things about the dietary choices that can lead to weight-loss success. In fact, by the time you finish this book, you'll be something of an expert on how to go from intention ("I want to lose weight") to achievement ("I lost 15 pounds and feel fantastic!"). To help you take stock of where you are now, spend a few minutes answering the following questions. Then, hang on to the answers because we'll be addressing each of these questions later in the book.

1. Do you skip breakfast as a rule?

2. If you do eat breakfast, is it filled with bread, potatoes, bacon or sausage, waffles, and pancakes?

3. Do you eat when you're not hungry?

4. Do you know when you're full?

5. If you eat at fast-food restaurants, do you opt for the double or triple burger with large fries and a soda?

6. Do you snack on nuts or nut butter out of the jar or can?

7. Do you eat while watching TV, driving, talking on your phone, or working at your desk and computer?

8. Are you the first one to begin eating your food when having a meal with others?

9. Do you eat everything on your plate for the benefit of the "starving children in Africa" because you learned to clean your plate as a child and not be wasteful?

10. Are raw fruits and raw or lightly cooked vegetables an infrequent part of your diet, or do you only eat them when they're bathed in butter, cream, or sugar?

11. Is working out a drag for you, a task that you can't seem to find the time for?

12. Do you eat meat more than three times per week?

13. Are you most likely to include sugary snacks and treats in your meal plan rather than fresh produce?

14. Do you think the portion sizes you are served at restaurants are overly large?

15. Do you believe you could change your lifestyle by losing weight using diet or exercise?

What You Gain When You Lose

We all want to look great. We want to be slim, sexy, and gorgeous. Dropping excess weight helps us to look good, that's for sure. But there are so many other important reasons to release the extra pounds we carry. If you're setting out on your weight-loss journey in hopes of looking better, that's fine. You'll get there. But I want you to think about your health, too, because weight loss can do some amazing things for your inside as well as your outside.

I know firsthand the toll that poor diet, a sedentary lifestyle, and a lot of extra weight can take on the human body. Growing up, I watched many members of my extended family, my neighborhood, and my community experience debilitating disability and early death because of what we now refer to as lifestyle diseases: heart disease, type 2 diabetes, cancer, stroke, peripheral vascular disease, and many others. And over the years, I've worked with thousands of patients and clients whose lives have been negatively affected by weight-related diseases. And let me tell you: When these people are on their deathbeds looking back at their lives, many of them wish they could go back and make changes.

Now is your time to change. Please don't wait until after you've had a heart attack, after you've had your foot amputated because of diabetic neuropathy, or after you've had part of your intestines removed because of advanced colorectal cancer. Use the F-15 Plan to make changes that can lower your risk of disability, disease, and early death. Do it now, before you're on your deathbed.

Making poor diet and exercise choices can profoundly increase your risk of developing three diseases that are among the top causes of death in the United States: diabetes, heart disease, and cancer. Let's look at how these three diseases are influenced by diet and exercise, because understanding what's at stake can have a big impact on your motivation to follow the F-15 Plan.

DIABETES: NOT SO SWEET

I talk a lot about diabetes in this book. Why? Diabetes robbed so many of my loved ones of their well-being. Aunts, uncles, cousins, and friends—I can't tell you how many of them have been affected by diabetes. It's afflicted so many of my clients, too. Diabetes is a terrible disease, and what's most painful of all is the fact that in too many cases, it can be prevented or controlled with diet and exercise.

(By the way, when I mention diabetes, I'm talking about type 2 diabetes, the kind that can be influenced by diet. Type 1 diabetes, which is also known as juvenile or insulin-dependent diabetes, is an autoimmune disorder that is not related to diet.)

Here are some things you should know about diabetes.

First, here's a quick explanation of blood sugar: When we eat food, our bodies turn it into glucose, or blood sugar, so we can use it for fuel. A hormone called insulin, which is manufactured by the pancreas, ushers glucose into our cells, where it is used to fuel the activities of everyday life. In people with diabetes, either their pancreas doesn't make enough insulin or their bodies resist the action of insulin. Because of this, too much glucose remains in the blood rather than being brought into cells, resulting in a situation known as high blood sugar, or high glucose. Having excess glucose in the blood can cause devastating damage to the body, and it can lead to complications such as heart disease, blindness, kidney damage, and loss of circulation that can result in amputation.

Now, the numbers: Some 29.1 million Americans have diabetes (that's about 1 out of every 11 people). Diabetes is the seventh leading cause of death in the United States. And about 8.1 million Americans have undiagnosed diabetes, which means they have diabetes but don't know it and aren't being treated for it. There are no cures for diabetes, but you can slow down its progress by keeping it under control. The best ways to do this are through diet, exercise, weight loss, and taking medication.

Before full-blown diabetes develops, most people have prediabetes. With prediabetes, blood sugar levels are higher than normal but not high enough to be considered diabetes. Approximately 86 million Americans—one in three people—have prediabetes, and an astonishing 90 percent don't know it. Here's the good news about prediabetes: If you have it, you can cut your risk of developing diabetes in half by making changes to your diet, activity level, and weight. If you have prediabetes and don't do anything about it, you have a 15 to 30 percent chance of developing diabetes within the next 5 years.

Your doctor can tell you for sure if you have diabetes or prediabetes using simple blood tests to measure your blood glucose level.

Q&A

DIABETES IN THE FAMILY

Q: **I have relatives on both sides of my family with diabetes. Does that mean I will get it? Is diabetes hereditary?**

A: Type 1 and type 2 diabetes do have genetic components. But that doesn't mean you're destined to develop them simply because they're in your family. Research suggests that other factors come into play that "turn on" diabetes genes. These factors include weight, exercise habits, and diet. So if you have diabetes in your family, you can fight back against any genetic predisposition by losing weight, eating a healthy diet, and exercising—in other words, by following the F-15 Plan and doing exactly what I'm telling you to do in this book! Multiple studies have found that when people take these steps, they can dramatically reduce their risk of developing diabetes, even if they have it in their family.

HEART DISEASE: OUR BIGGEST KILLER

The facts are chilling: Heart disease is the number-one cause of death in America. More than 610,000 Americans die of heart disease each year (that's one in four deaths). In the United States, someone dies of a heart disease–related event every *minute*.

That's just the start of it. Statistics show that about half of all Americans have at least one of the three main risk factors for heart disease: high blood pressure, high LDL cholesterol, and smoking. And many more Americans are in danger of developing or dying from heart disease because they have other major risk factors, including diabetes, overweight or obesity, poor diet, physical inactivity, or excessive alcohol use.

Statistics show that about half of all Americans have at least one of the three main risk factors for heart disease: high blood pressure, high LDL cholesterol, and smoking.

I could keep going with facts and statistics like these, but I think you get the idea: Heart disease is a huge problem. But the good news is that adopting a healthy diet and exercise program such as the F-15 Plan can help lower heart disease risk. That's because my eating plan addresses nearly all of the major risk factors for heart disease. In addition to losing weight and improving diet, people who follow the tenants of the F-15 Plan have the potential to lower their blood pressure and LDL cholesterol and to reduce their risk of developing diabetes. It's a win-win situation.

Simply losing weight lowers heart disease risk. When you drop excess pounds, your body is better able to circulate its blood more efficiently. There is less strain on your heart. And as your weight goes down, so do your chances of developing diabetes, high blood pressure, and other conditions that increase heart disease risk.

If you're worried about your heart, stick with me: The F-15 Plan will help chip away at your risk of becoming one of those disturbing statistics.

CANCER: A GROWING CONCERN

Being overweight or obese raises the risk of developing certain kinds of cancer. According to the National Cancer Institute, obesity is associated with a higher risk of cancer of the esophagus, pancreas, colon and rectum, breast (after menopause), endometrium (lining of the uterus), kidney, thyroid, and bladder. Researchers estimate that 4 percent of cancers in men and 7 percent of cancers in women are due to obesity, although for some types, such as endometrial cancer and esophageal adenocarcinoma, obesity plays a part in as many as 40 percent of cases.

And as the number of obese people in America increases, so will the number of obesity-related cancers.

As with the other diseases I've mentioned, you can reduce the risk by losing extra weight. In fact, even modest weight loss can bring about change. Cancer and weight are connected in several ways that we know about—and probably more ways that we haven't yet figured out. For one, fat tissue produces extra estrogen, which has been associated with breast cancer and some other types of cancer. Excess fat can also impact the levels of certain hormones, tumor growth regulators, and inflammation, which play a part in some forms of cancer development.

There is no need to go into more detail than that; suffice to say that overall cancer risk increases with excess weight and is reduced when that weight is lost. Stick with me and the F-15 Plan, and you'll be better positioned to stave off many health risks.

Q&A

A BOOST OF GOOD HEALTH

Q: **Will following the F-15 Plan improve my health?**

A: The F-15 Plan absolutely has the potential to boost your health and to reduce your risk of disease! Once you start losing weight, your chances of developing various health problems can go down. For example, current research suggests that losing the weight may help reduce your risk for the following (hold on to your hat, because this list is long!): Alzheimer's disease, amputations, asthma, back pain, certain kinds of blindness, cervical cancer, circulatory problems, colorectal cancer, endometrial cancer, esophageal cancer, gallbladder cancer, gallbladder disease, gastroesophageal reflux disease (GERD), gestational diabetes, heart attack, heart failure, high blood pressure, infections, infertility, irregular heartbeat, joint diseases (osteoarthritis, gout), kidney cancer, kidney disease, leukemia, liver cancer, liver disease, metabolic syndrome, miscarriage and stillbirth, multiple myeloma, nerve damage, non-Hodgkin's lymphoma, ovarian cancer, pancreatic cancer, postmenopausal breast cancer, premature birth, prostate cancer, sexual impotence, sleep apnea, stress urinary incontinence, stroke, and thyroid cancer.

In the Next Chapter:
Changing Your Mindset

Now you have an idea of what to expect from me, from this book, from the F-15 Plan and how we can work together to help you shed excess pounds and lower your risk of three diseases that are major causes of death and disability for people who are overweight or obese.

Now we're going to spend a little time looking at the ways in which you think about food and weight. Believe it or not, it's your mind—not your stomach—that most often interferes with your intentions to eat a healthy diet. But don't worry: I have created an easy, step-by-step plan that will help you shift into a healthy, successful F-15 Mindset. I'll tell you all about it in Chapter 2.

Chapter 2

PLANNING FOR SUCCESS: ADOPTING THE F-15 MINDSET

There is no amount of cake, ice cream,
potato chips, or any food that can fill
the emptiness of despair.
—Dr. Ro

The F-15 Plan combines several important approaches to weight loss: diet, meal planning, exercise, and stress reduction, among others. But before we talk about the specifics of the F-15 Plan, I want us to sit down and have a heart-to-heart about something that's even more important than what you eat or how you move.

Wait a minute, you may be thinking. The F-15 Plan is a diet plan. Shouldn't we be talking about food? Don't worry—we'll get to that. But this chapter is about how to plan for success, and if I've learned nothing else during my many years working with all different kinds of clients, it's this: Weight-loss success starts in your head. Sure, what happens on your plate is tremendously important. And the exercise habits you develop make a huge difference, as well. But the people who are most successful at shedding excess weight are the ones who start doing so by changing the way they *think*, not just the way they eat. It's not about what goes on in your stomach, my friend. It's all about what happens in your mind. The easiest way to lose weight and keep it off for good is to develop a mindset that supports, encourages, and enables the choices that lead to weight-loss success.

I call this the F-15 Mindset.

The ways in which you think about food and weight and your understanding of what drives you to eat, as well as how you respond to your emotions, all play a huge role in weight gain and weight loss. It's not enough just to change the way you eat and move. Unless you make some important shifts in how you think, weight loss will elude you. Believe me—I know what I'm talking about. Adopting the F-15 Mindset changes everything.

What exactly is the F-15 Mindset? It's a set of mindful strategies that help you to restructure your thought patterns, shifting them in directions that support rather than sabotage you. The F-15 Mindset offers a whole new way of thinking about food.

In this chapter, we'll identify thought patterns that work against you. Then we'll restructure them, spinning them into a positive direction to channel your mind's energy into a positive force for weight-loss success. In sports, athletes talk about the importance of having their head in the game; they say games are won in their minds, rather than on the fields or courts. The same is true of the weight-loss "game." In my experience, nothing is a better predictor of success than having the right mindset.

So pull up a chair. Put up your feet and get comfy. Let's take a look at what's going on in your head, and I'll show you exactly how you can develop the super-successful F-15 Mindset.

> *What exactly is the F-15 Mindset? It's a set of mindful strategies that help you to restructure your thought patterns, shifting them in directions that support rather than sabotage you. The F-15 Mindset offers a whole new way of thinking about food.*

Shift into Thin Thinking

When people start a weight-loss plan, they spend a lot of time thinking about changing the way they eat. That's definitely important—after all, if you keep on eating the same exact foods and quantities, you're not going to lose any weight. You have to make some changes to the types of food you eat as well as the serving sizes you heap onto your plate.

The same goes for the way you think. To change the way you *eat*, you have to change the way you *think* about eating. This reminds me of a quote from Albert Einstein: "Insanity is doing the same thing over and over again and expecting different results." That's what we do with our dietary thinking. We expect somehow to lose weight even when we keep eating the same foods over and over again and thinking about food in the same way. That's insane! I refer to this as fat thinking vs. thin thinking. You're probably engaging in lots of *fat thinking*, and I'm going to help you reframe your thought processes so you can shift into *thin thinking*.

What's fat thinking? It's eating like you used to eat rather than the way you ought to eat. It's eating when you're not really hungry and sabotaging yourself by making poor choices rather than great choices.

What's fat thinking? It's eating like you used to eat, rather than the way you ought to eat. It's eating when you're not really hungry and sabotaging yourself by making poor choices rather than great choices. Here's an example. You're having dinner at the home of a relative who served you large portions of her delicious cooking. You're deciding how much of those delicious ribs and coleslaw to eat. With fat thinking, you clean your plate, but with thin thinking, you eat only what fits into your day's eating plan, and you leave the rest on your plate. It may not seem like much, but you can save yourself hundreds of calories per meal simply by resigning your membership in the Clean Plate Club. Fat thinking tells you to eat everything on your plate; thin thinking guides you to leave some behind.

Here's another example. Say you're feeling really stressed: You're behind on a big work assignment, or you just received some bad news. If you're engaging in fat thinking, you'll head for the kitchen, grab a pint of ice cream from the freezer, and soothe your stressful feelings with food. That's fat thinking, and all it ever does is make you fatter than you want to be. Thin thinking is the opposite: When you are stressed and feel yourself being called to the kitchen, you take a deep breath, decide you're going to do some thin thinking, and look for other ways to reduce your stressful feelings, like going for a walk, calling a friend, spending 15 minutes meditating, or playing some really loud music and dancing to the beat.

To get a really good feeling of what thin thinking looks like, spend some time with your thin friends. Pay close attention to how they react to the ups and downs of life. Watch the choices they make. I have a thin friend who will take a few bites of birthday cake and then just stop eating. This used to amaze me (who can walk away from half a slice of birthday cake?). I asked her about it once, and she just shrugged her shoulders. "That's all I ate because that's all I needed." Now that, my friends, is thin thinking.

Shifting from fat to thin thinking is a process. In fact, you can start making small changes right away. Mindfulness plays an important role in thin thinking. If you make your choices automatically, without stopping to think, you're much more likely to give in to fat thinking. But if you slow yourself down a bit to be really mindful of every decision you're making, you will make better choices. Mindful thinking takes practice, but it's worth the effort because it will help you transform your fat thinking into thin thinking and ultimately transform your body and your life.

Look at it this way: You want to make choices that fit the body you want, not the body you have. Going to the movies and ordering a big tub of buttered popcorn and a giant cup of sugary soda is fat thinking; it's a decision that reflects the body you have. Bringing along a small bag of air-popped popcorn from home and washing it down with a bottle of water is thin thinking; it's a choice that will lead you to the body you want.

Every time you are at a decision point with food—which, by the way, happens more than 200 times a day for most Americans—stop and take a few breaths. Ask yourself: What is the best choice for the body I want? What choice will keep me stuck with the body I have? Be honest with yourself. Trust me, lying won't get you anywhere at all.

Here's another way to wrap your head around all of this. Compare it with money. We are all very aware of the idea of being on a financial budget. We know we need X amount of dollars for the rent or mortgage every month, a certain amount for the gas bill and the electric bill, a certain amount for groceries—you know how that goes. All month long, we keep our budgets in mind. We know how much we have available to spend on this or that. And as we make choices about making purchases, we stop and think about whether those purchases are worthwhile. If a pair of shoes costs $150, we stop and think about it before buying. We ask ourselves: Do I need these shoes? Do I have $150 to spend on fashion? Are these shoes worth $150? Should I put the purchase off until another time? Should I skip the $150 shoes and just get by with the ones I already have?

The same process should happen when we're deciding to spend *calories*. Say you're in the kitchen, you're hungry, and there's a bag of tortilla chips sitting on the counter. Stop and think about it before you eat them up. Ask yourself: Do I need these chips? Do I have 300 or 400 calories in my day's calorie budget to spend on these chips? Are they worth all those calories? Should I toss them in the trash and spend my calories more wisely on a nutritious snack that is packed with protein and fiber and has far fewer calories? When you think about it this way, you're very likely to say to yourself, "Ditch those chips!" That's what I call engaging in thin thinking, because you're fully aware of your calorie budget, and you make choices that fit your goals and the realities of your life.

Bottom line? Each time you are presented with the opportunity to eat, ask yourself if the calories are worth it to you. Ask yourself if you even want the food. You will have many opportunities presented to you, whether you notice that someone hasn't finished her plate or that there is an extra serving of pasta or chocolate cake on the table. Just because it's there doesn't mean you have to eat it.

Emotional Eating:
What Are You Hungry For?

As you are probably well aware, emotional eating and cravings are two giant wrecking balls that can smash up even the best-designed, most well-intentioned meal plans. Based on my experience, emotional eating and cravings are the top reasons that weight-loss plans fail.

It's one thing to begin a savvy meal plan that puts the right foods on your plate and gets the results you want. Certainly, being mindful of what you're eating is an important part of the process. But as I tell my clients, at some point we've got to get to the bottom of what's really eating you.

That's why it makes sense to look at emotional eating and cravings now, before you immerse yourself in the F-15 Plan. Once you have a full understanding of what causes emotional eating and cravings, you can make better choices when these feelings hit. Let's start with the basics. We experience two kinds of hunger: physical hunger and emotional hunger—in other words, hunger in our bodies and hunger in our minds. Physical hunger occurs when our bodies require the energy from food in order to continue functioning well. Physical hunger is an actual physiological sensation that occurs in a predictable, physiological way.

Picture yourself eating breakfast. After waking up hungry, you sit down to a bowl of yogurt, some berries, and a cup of coffee. As soon as you begin to eat and food travels from your mouth to your stomach, your body starts to respond. The hormone leptin, which is known as the satiety hormone, is released into your blood. As you continue eating, leptin levels rise. When they hit a certain point, your hunger subsides.

After breakfast, you begin your day. You feel satiated by your breakfast and don't feel hungry. But during the hours that follow, your leptin levels begin to plummet. When they become low enough, your body reacts by releasing the hormone ghrelin, which is known as the hunger hormone. Ghrelin triggers your hunger for more food. Your stomach begins to contract, creating hunger pangs that are true physical manifestations of your body's physiological need for food. After having something to eat, your leptin levels hit a certain point, your hunger goes away, and you stop eating. During the hours that follow, leptin levels go down, and when it's time to eat again, your body releases the hormone ghrelin, which triggers appetite and hunger for more food.

Unfortunately, if you're overweight or obese, your body becomes less able to "read" the messages sent by hormones such as leptin. And studies suggest leptin levels may be low overall in obese people. When the leptin cut-off mechanism becomes less effective, people are less able to realize that they're full and should stop eating. Problems like this can also arise for people whose insulin response is off-kilter, as it often is with people who have diabetes, pre-diabetes, or insulin resistance.

Lots of other processes are involved in the sensation of hunger. Blood sugar levels fall, and various other neurochemicals and hormones tell your body that it's time for your next meal. Physical hunger is one of the strongest drives that the human body experiences.

Hunger in Your Mind

Not all hunger is physical, however. We also experience emotional hunger, which I define as a desire to eat that is not connected to physical hunger. It is hunger that originates in your brain rather than your belly. Emotional hunger is a powerful force: Research suggests that as much as three-quarters of our food choices—about 188 daily choices—are driven by emotional rather than physical hunger.

Emotional hunger is caused not by an empty stomach but by feelings that create discomfort: stress, anxiety, loneliness, boredom, impatience, anger, and frustration, to name a few. When we feel these difficult emotions, we become uncomfortable, and we want them to go away; we want to calm our stress, reduce our anxiety, or feel less bored, impatient, frustrated, or angry. Rather than doing the work needed to face up to what causes these emotions—for example, having a heart-to-heart conversation with your spouse after an argument—we reach for food instead.

Positive feelings can trigger emotional hunger, too. Many of my clients have a "let's celebrate with food" reaction to anything good that happens, big or small. This is fine to some extent; I am not going to tell you to skip that celebratory dinner after you get a raise at work. But happy eating has to have a limit. I've learned that it is just as important to learn to discipline our pleasure as it is to discipline our disappointment. A writer friend of mine got into the habit of eating an M&M's candy after each successful paragraph she wrote—and she wondered why she gained 20 pounds with every book she finished.

EATING TO CURE EMOTIONAL PAIN

Emotional hunger often leads to a food craving, which is an intense desire to eat a certain food. Researchers have found that food cravings are one of the major reasons people overeat, gain weight, and fail at losing weight. It is my experience that when cravings hit, my clients are not necessarily hungry for food. Rather, they are looking to meet an emotional need or satisfy some kind of longing. They're eating to cure an ill—to soothe an emotional emptiness. Solving emotional problems can be difficult and time-consuming, so they turn to food instead (for example, it's much easier to scarf down a pizza than to try to figure out how to save your failing marriage). And when you consider how many people have been taught from childhood that food is the answer to curing their emotional ills, it's understandable that so many adults turn to food as an elixir. Think back to when you were a child; many of us grew up in a home in which food was offered as comfort or a reward and perhaps withheld as punishment. No wonder we associate food with emotional support.

Researchers have found that for people who experience cravings, eating the foods they crave can actually bring about changes in brain activity that can make them feel better. For example, eating chocolate can release brain chemicals that soothe, relax, and provide pleasure. Unfortunately, although eating chocolate whenever you feel unhappy may make you feel better for a minute or two, it backfires afterward when you feel bad about going off your eating plans or when you gain weight. It's better to learn to cope with cravings than to allow them to rule your world.

It's not surprising that turning to food for emotional solace can bring on such bad feelings, including guilt. And for my clients, comparison to others and the feeling of not measuring up further exacerbates the remorse they feel. Take my word for it: You are never going to find happiness by comparing yourself with other people. The fact is no one can be a better you! You've got that part on lock. There will always be loads of people who are better looking than you, thinner than you, richer than you, more successful than you (depending on how you define success, but you get my point). And, of course, there are people who aren't doing as well as you, but who compares themselves to people in worse positions? No one does. Instead, most people fall into the trap of looking up and wondering why they're down so much further than all the people who seem to be doing so much better than they are. It's true: Comparison is the thief of your joy. It is a losing proposition to compare yourself to another person, but by the same token, there is no one on the planet who can do or be a better you. That's why I want you to compare yourself only to yourself. Forget about the other people. As you lose weight, put up a picture of yourself on your refrigerator—your better self, when you were at a healthier weight. That's what you can strive for! You want to be the best version of yourself, always! It is the one thing at which you will never fail.

No matter how hard I work, for example, I'm never going to look like Naomi Campbell. Never! So if I try to do that, all I'm going to be is disappointed. Instead of wishing for the impossible, I remind myself: There is no other Dr. Ro. I can't be anyone else, and I don't want to be anyone else. But I can be the best version of me that there has ever been. When I set out to lose weight for the last time, I had a picture of myself from college. I made copies and hung them everywhere—on my bedroom mirror, in the bathroom, in my car, everywhere! That is what I wanted to look and feel like—my younger, healthier, more energetic best self. I knew I'd never have the body of a 20-year-old again, but I also knew that by doing my best every day, I could move as close to my goal as possible. That drove me to the point of a 30-pound weight-loss goal. Keeping pictures of when you were your most productive, healthy, fit, and beautiful (or handsome) self on your phone, tablet, fridge, mirror, or any place you frequent on a daily basis as a reminder just might motivate you, too.

No matter what triggers your cravings and emotional eating, you'll do best if you take control of it. Otherwise, it will control you, and you'll be unable to succeed with the F-15 Plan or any other weight-loss program.

Much More Than Fuel

Food is the fuel that runs our bodies. But because of the emotional connections we have with food, it is so much more than fuel. We celebrate, mourn, and medicate with food. What do I mean by that? Well, take a look at your own life.

We celebrate holidays and special occasions with food. Think of cake and ice cream on birthdays. And think of the elaborate holiday meals we

THE ENGINEERED CRAVING

If you are interested in learning more about how big corporations use the science of craving to sell more food, I suggest you read the book *Cooked: A Natural History of Transformation*, by Michael Pollan. In it, Pollan talks about how food manufacturers use sugar, salt, and fat in ways that entice us to keep eating more food and calories than we need. It is truly eye-opening!

In response to these commercial machinations, Pollan advocates for, as I do, more mindful home cooking with whole, fresh foods. Home cooking doesn't have to be labor-intensive; you can focus on quick, simple recipes that use healthy amounts of inexpensive ingredients (like the recipes in this book, for example). Instead of spending time, money, and energy on elaborate meals, Pollan suggests, as I did in my first book, *Dr. Ro's Ten Secrets to Livin' Healthy*, making meals social, sacred times where the emphasis is on relationships rather than on high-calorie dishes. I couldn't agree more!

eat to the point of exhaustion, feeling so overstuffed that the top button on our pants or skirt has to be loosened. We also mourn with food. When we're upset about something, one of the first things we do is head for the refrigerator. And think about the huge repasts we set out after funerals!

Worst of all, we self-medicate with food. I consider food to be the number-one drug of our time. Think about the times you (or someone you may know—I don't judge) drowned your sorrows in a pint of Ben & Jerry's ice cream to get over someone who couldn't love you the way your heart needed. Or the time your boss or kids made you so angry that nothing would do except devouring a big bag of something crunchy. The point is, all of these behaviors are direct responses to our emotional need for food beyond what our bodies actually require. These are all factors that have in part led to the dreaded statistic of two-thirds of America being overweight or obese. But, you know, I'm a naturally optimistic person. So I will always see the glass as half full. These statistics don't bother me because I know that if you want to change this, you can. You are strong, you are smart, and simply by picking up this book, you are taking action. You can break free of emotional eating, break free of all the habits that are keeping you in an unhealthy place. You can make the changes to live a healthier, happier life. I know you can! To help you, I've created the following five-step plan to cope with emotional eating and cravings. It will help you learn how to stop letting your emotional hunger get the best of you.

Dr. Ro's Emotional Eating Plan: How to Understand What's Eating You

Ready to start dealing with the various kinds of feelings and automatic reactions that trigger emotional eating? Use my step-by-step plan to understand what's eating you and how to restructure the thinking behind the eating.

STEP #1: TAKE A MINDFUL MOMENT

We respond automatically to feelings of hunger. We feel hungry, we go to the refrigerator, we grab a piece of cheese or a tub of Ben & Jerry's, and we gobble it up—all without thinking or analyzing our feelings or actions. By slowing that process down, you can begin to take control of emotional hunger.

The first step toward reducing emotional eating is stopping yourself anytime you feel hungry, analyzing your feelings, and determining whether your hunger is originating from your stomach or your mind. Instead of reflexively running off to the kitchen, I want you to take a few minutes to think about your hunger and determine whether its origin is emotional or physical. This isn't difficult, although it does take a commitment to mindfulness, a promise to yourself that you'll slow down and look at your feelings and actions almost as an outsider would. Ask yourself: What do I *really* want? Do I really need food, or something else? When you experience a feeling of hunger, don't just run to get something to eat. Instead, stop yourself. Sit down, close your eyes, and ask yourself a few questions. What am I feeling? Do I feel physically hungry? Am I having hunger pangs? Has it been 2 to 3 hours or just a few minutes since I ate last? Ask yourself about the nature of your hunger. Did it come on quickly or has your stomach been rumbling for a while? Emotional hunger tends to come on quickly.

Ask yourself about the nature of your hunger. Did it come on quickly or has your stomach been rumbling for a while? Emotional hunger tends to come on quickly.

When you have a craving, a couple of things happen. You anticipate positive reinforcement when you eat—that is, you expect to feel better—and you also expect to eliminate negative feelings, such as sadness, anger, or loneliness. However, those good feelings may not occur at all, or they may be immediately overridden by even more negative feelings, such as guilt and shame.

If you realize you're not physically hungry, take a minute to think about what's going on in your head. Are you experiencing a difficult emotion? Did something occur recently that provoked an emotional response, such as an argument with your boss, a rejection from a business contact, or a frustrating exchange with a friend? Are you frustrated, angry, or annoyed? Are you happy, relieved, or joyful? Are you bored or lonely? Analyze your feelings and really try to label them so you can understand what's behind them and the action you've become accustomed to taking when you feel them.

Now, ask yourself what you're thinking of eating. Are you answering the call of the chocolate bar you tucked away on a high shelf? Or are you thinking you'll grab an apple? This is important because emotional hunger tends to cause cravings for specific foods—such as chocolate cake, cookies, or salty snacks—rather than healthier choices, such as fruits, vegetables, or a handful of nuts. When you're physically hungry, you're more likely to look for your next healthy meal or snack rather than an indulgence.

Looking at pictures of foods triggers cravings (why do you think advertisers use such delicious-looking photography?). As you work to cope with cravings, try to cut back on visual-craving creators, such as TV ads. If you're watching your favorite show, jump onto the treadmill, jog in place, or do squats, lunges, or triceps dips on a chair instead of viewing commercials. Pay close attention to the external triggers that influence your desire for food.

After spending a couple of mindful moments examining the source of your hunger, you'll be better prepared to make a thoughtful choice about whether and what to eat. But before you do that, I want you to grab a pen (or your smartphone) and take Step 2.

STEP #2: PUT IT IN WRITING

Keeping a food journal is a crucial part of the F-15 Plan. Use whatever format you like for a food journal—a notebook, your smartphone, a spreadsheet on your laptop. It doesn't matter what you use as long as you note a few things, including the time of day, a description of your hunger, and what you're feeling and why you're feeling it. The "why" is important and, believe it or not, could date back to an experience you had years ago but never identified as a connection to food for you.

We'll talk more about food journals later in the book. But for now, I want you to start keeping a "cravings journal." When you find yourself craving food, take a minute to jot down the answers to these questions: What am I craving? What am I feeling? Why am I feeling this feeling? How might I satisfy my craving without bingeing on a high-calorie food?

Keep your cravings journal close at hand because you'll use it during the following steps, as well.

STEP #3: MAKE A DECISION

Now that you've analyzed your hunger and decided whether its source is emotional or physical, you can make a better choice about whether, and what, to eat. If your hunger is physical, you may be able to put it off for a while, accepting the fact that, yes, you do feel physically hungry but it's okay to feel that way and wait until your next meal to satisfy that hunger. Or you may realize you're overdue for your next meal or snack, so it's time to head for the kitchen to prepare something that fits right in to your new F-15 Plan. Those are two good ways to respond to physical hunger.

If your hunger is emotional, it may be harder to put off. Emotional hunger is more gnawing and persistent than physical hunger. Ignoring it sometimes works, but as someone who has longed for ice cream, I can tell you that the "just say no" strategy doesn't always work. But you don't want to give in and inhale 600 calories worth of your fantasy food. Instead, try these alternatives.

Eat a substitute food. Say you're craving something salty, spicy, and crunchy, such as tortilla chips, and all you can think about is having a bag of Doritos. It's possible that eating something else salty, spicy, and crunchy will suffice—maybe a few pieces of celery sprinkled with taco seasoning or air-popped popcorn dusted with chili powder. If you're craving something sweet, a piece of fruit or an F-15 dessert (see my Banana Nice Cream recipe, page 192) may do the trick. Other good cravings chasers for creamy, savory, and sweet foods include these healthy alternatives: mashed boiled cauliflower with low-fat cheese, fat-free sour cream, or fat-free cream cheese (instead of mashed potatoes); grab-n-go sugar-free pudding or Jell-O cups with fruit; a baked apple topped with cinnamon and chopped walnuts; or watermelon chunks sprinkled with chili powder.

Do a substitute activity. Sometimes, an alternative activity can fill the emotional need that stands behind your craving. Need comfort? Go to a park or some other lovely space, even if it's to your bathroom for an herbal-scented, candlelit bath. Feeling isolated? Stroke your pet or read an affirming passage that inspires and builds you up. I find that feelings of loneliness and isolation can be easily chased away by doing good deeds for others. You may be surprised to find how quickly and completely you can heal your pain by doing something good for someone else in need. Feeling bored and lethargic? Try going for a run or walk instead of eating a handful of cookies. Feeling superstressed or tense? Bring stress levels down with activities that match the intensity of your emotions. Go for a jog or power walk, dance to loud upbeat music, beat on a pillow, kickbox, or spar to release tension. You could try aromatherapy. One study found that sniffing jasmine aromas helped some people curtail chocolate cravings. Even playing a video game may help. Cravings are visual, and according to a study published in 2014 in the journal *Appetite*, visual games like Tetris help distract people from food cravings by replacing visual images in their minds of food. In the study, food cravings in volunteers who played video games were reduced by 24 percent compared to those who engaged in no visually distracting behavior. According to researchers, the mental processes we experience as we think about food cravings can be overridden by the mental processes needed to focus on a video game. Eureka! There's hope for the chocoholic in each of us yet!

Have just a nibble. Let's face it: Some food cravings just won't go away unless you give in. Deprivation sometimes works, but often it backfires, and instead of having nothing, you binge on a large amount of some food not included in your meal plan. When that's the case, contain the possible damage by having a small amount of the food you crave. Scientists say that we start feeling satisfied after just three or four bites. Indulge in just a small amount of the food you crave. Eat it slowly and mindfully, allowing yourself to enjoy it fully. Stop after three bites, and see how you feel. That small amount may very well chase your craving away, assuming you really consumed the advice I gave you in the last few paragraphs about mindful eating and thinking before you leap.

Once you decide how to respond to your craving, grab your cravings journal and write down the choice you made. I can tell—you're ready to make better choices already aren't you? Yessss! You are so getting there!

STEP #4: DO A GUT CHECK

Around 15 minutes after you eat, take a moment to examine your feelings on the choice you made about whether/what to eat. Do you feel satisfied and peaceful? Or do you feel guilty and shameful? Did you continue eating when you were full, or did you stop after consuming a reasonable amount?

If after 15 minutes you feel unhappy with the choice you made, reflect on how you might have acted differently. But do it with a positive spin. Remember that the goal here is to learn from your mistakes, to take lessons away from your experience. I do not want you to feel angry at yourself or to beat yourself up for making a poor choice; all that will do is bring you down and lead you to even more emotional eating. If you feel you made a mistake, acknowledge it and learn from it. Make a note in your food journal of any lessons you may have learned from the experience. And then, move on, knowing that the experience can help you the next time you feel emotional hunger. Again, this is a process. In order to master it, you will have to walk it out until you get it right. The length of time it takes for the process to unfold is determined by you alone. I believe in you, and I need you to believe, too!

STEP #5: DEAL WITH THE FEELINGS

Now it's time to take a look at the feelings that triggered your emotional hunger and to brainstorm a few nonfood responses that you can use the next time you experience those feelings. This may be a simple step—for example, if you conclude that being tired triggered your craving, you may decide to start going to bed a bit earlier or to take a nap when the feeling returns.

If the emotion behind your craving is more complex, you may need to think about a more long-term solution. For example, if stress about a bad relationship is pushing you into the kitchen, you may need to consider getting counseling or ending the relationship. If a horrible boss drives you to the comfort that chocolate provides, it may be time for a meeting with human resources or even thinking about a new job. And if depression or anxiety causes cravings, it may make sense for you to see your doctor or a therapist who can help you manage these emotional problems. Whatever you determine the best solution for you to be, know this: You must deal with the problems that cause you misery. You deserve to live a life unhampered by a dysfunctional relationship with food exacerbated by unhealthy relationships with other people or yourself.

Work on catching your uncomfortable feelings before they take root. Recognize the resentment and feelings of inadequacy as they begin and then separate in your mind your true self from the negative voice in your head. When problems can't be immediately solved, turn to positive distractions that take your mind away from what irks you. Take that writing or knitting class you've been meaning to get around to. Volunteer at a women's shelter or a children's nursery. Drive a senior citizen to the doctor or run errands for someone who can't do it for herself. You'd be surprised by how good these acts of kindness will make you feel.

Likewise, filling your soul with spiritual nourishment may take away some of your cravings for food. When you find greater meaning in your own life, food moves to the back of the room and off center stage. Allowing yourself to be nourished by a relationship with God, the love of your family, or other soul-satisfying gifts enables you to make food just a source of nourishment again. Gaining control of your food cravings and learning to manage emotional eating will help you to develop a much-needed healthy and functional relationship with food, as opposed to the dysfunctional relationship that most emotional and stress eaters live with every day.

Whatever you do, keep in mind that if you work toward solving the root problems behind your emotional need to eat, the cravings will begin to subside. My clients too often blame themselves for giving in to food cravings, beating themselves up for not having enough willpower to say no. But when it comes to emotional eating, it's not necessarily about willpower. It's about finding ways to cope with the emotions that lead you to food.

Q&A

CONSTANT CRAVINGS

Q: **My friends and I all seem to crave the same kinds of foods. Is this true for most people?**

A: Yes—we all tend to crave fatty foods that are either salty or sugary. In fact, researchers have identified the following as the most commonly craved foods: cheese, chocolate, pasta, red meat, salty snacks (popcorn, pretzels), fried potatoes (potato chips, french fries), comfort foods and casseroles (macaroni and cheese, chicken and rice casserole), foods associated with your childhood (chocolate chip cookies, mom's chicken noodle soup), foods associated with your culture (fried chicken, ribs, tacos, lasagna), ice cream, soda, spicy foods, and candy.

CLUES IN YOUR CRAVINGS

If you're not sure which emotion is causing your craving, think about this: For some people, the type of emotion that triggers a desire for food also influences the kind of food that's being craved. For example, if you can't stop thinking about having a giant Frappuccino or a tall glass of sweet iced tea, the cause may be boredom or lack of energy. Your mind wants to get revved up, so you crave energy-boosting, caffeine-filled treats. Here are some other foods that are sometimes linked to specific emotions.

Sweets: Sugar stimulates the release of the brain chemical dopamine, which mediates feelings of pleasure in the brain. And sugar and fat can help lower your blood levels of the stress hormone cortisol. If you're craving sweets, you may be feeling sad or bored, in need of some pleasure and happiness. Instead of sweets, try doing something fun, such as watching a funny movie or connecting with a fun friend.

Chocolate: Often referred to as the food of the gods, chocolate is satisfying in many ways—its luscious smell, its creamy taste, the way it feels when it melts on the tongue. Chocolate delivers pleasure and satisfaction, and it can trigger the release of the same brain chemicals that are produced during sex. You may think of chocolate when you are hungry for sensual pleasure in your life. Spending time with your honey may help reduce your desire for chocolate.

Cheese: Dairy foods contain amino acids that stimulate the release of serotonin, a feel-good brain chemical that soothes and relaxes. If you're hankering for a grilled cheese sandwich, pizza, or a huge slab of lasagna, you may be feeling stressed or anxious. A few minutes of meditation may chase away your desire for cheese.

Fatty foods: Full of calories, fat fills your belly up when it's empty—and for some people, it can help fill emotional emptiness, as well. You may crave fat when you're feeling lonely, bored, unchallenged, or sad. Hanging out with friends, starting a new project, or even doing a crossword puzzle may help you avoid high-fat binges.

Crunchy foods: Eating chips, cheese curls, buttery caramel corn, and other crunchy foods can help you release feelings of anger, tension, regret, bitterness, or frustration. Instead of chowing down on crunchy junk, try chewing up celery, carrots, and other healthier crunches such as nuts instead. Or snack on air-popped popcorn with Cajun seasoning, Butter Buds, or low-fat cheese sprinkles.

Fried foods: A desire for crunchy, fried foods (fried chicken or fish, french fries, corn curls) can also be a sign that you are looking for excitement. Instead of eating, try doing something that's really out there for you—sign up for sky diving lessons, take up a new sport, or try that new online dating service you've heard good things about.

Creamy foods: Hot cocoa with whipped cream, cream cheese, pudding, and other creamy foods represent comfort and soothing, and you may crave them when you feel like the world has been beating you up a bit. Instead of giving in and having creamy, high-calorie foods, try sharing your feelings with a friend or taking a hot bath.

Hot or cold foods: Your desire for soup, hot cocoa, café au lait, or even a superspicy burrito may simply mean you're cold rather than hungry. Likewise, your interest in ice cream or other frozen treats may just be your reaction to a rise in mercury. Instead of eating, try a change of temperature; wrap yourself up in a thick blanket if you're cold, or turn up the AC if you're hot.

Carbohydrates: Eating high-carb foods—such as bread, pasta, cookies, and cake—provides comfort. That's because carbs boost brain levels of serotonin, a chemical that soothes you. You may go for high-carb foods when you feel depressed, tired, or upset and in need of soothing. Instead of loading up on carbs, look for other ways to comfort yourself. Take a nap, listen to relaxing music, go for a walk by a lake, or give your mom or someone you love and trust a call.

Remember, everyone has cravings; they are completely normal. In studies conducted at Tufts University, researchers found that 91 percent of people experience food cravings. And the more you weigh, the more likely you are to crave high-calorie foods. Because cravings are a normal part of life, it's unrealistic to expect them just to go away. Tufts researchers found that even after 6 months of following a weight-loss eating plan, 94 percent of study participants continued to have cravings. Your best bet is to work with them. Get to know them. Understand them and create strategies to cope with them. That's the way to gain control over urges—any urges that lead to behaviors that you don't want—and instead lay the foundation for behaviors that get you to your goals.

IT'S OKAY TO BE TRULY HUNGRY

When you're thinking about cravings and hunger, try to keep this in mind: It's okay to be hungry. In my one-on-one work with clients, I find that many of them are irrationally afraid of getting physically hungry. While I do recommend that you eat every 3 or 4 hours, making sure to include a protein source, don't worry too much if you are running late and can't eat—being hungry won't hurt you. Often my clients carry food around as if they're preparing for a famine, with chocolate-coated granola bars in their purses, crackers in their glove compartments, and cookies in their desk drawers. Many of them eat proactively in order to prevent themselves from ever feeling hunger pangs. This isn't necessary. When I suggest that they start allowing themselves to feel hungry, they worry about how it will play out for them—but when I remind them that what they've been doing hasn't been working for them, they usually open their minds to it.

It's okay to let yourself get hungry. Not ravenous, because that's usually when out-of-control eating occurs. But a few hunger pangs here and there are fine. When you get them, notice how they feel, and remind yourself that they won't destroy you.

When you feel physical hunger, don't always run for something to eat. Believe it or not, the signals to the brain that communicate hunger are the same ones the brain receives for thirst. Try drinking a tall glass of water, and wait for a few minutes to determine whether you were actually thirsty. If that doesn't satisfy your urge to grab food, just try to put it out of your mind until it's time for your next meal or snack. Eventually, you'll become less uncomfortable with the feelings of physical hunger. And as you lose weight, you'll feel hunger pangs less often. On the F-15 Plan, you will be eating every 3 to 4 hours, depending on your calorie needs.

QUESTION YOUR CRAVINGS

Long before the piece of double-chocolate cake touches your lips, you've eaten it over and over again and remembered what it made you feel like each time you had it before—in your mind. Cravings most often begin in the mind. So before you actually *taste* the food that you crave, you actually eat it in your mind. Therein lies your opportunity to take control of your cravings and take back your own power over an emotional appetite. Think about it. You have the power—in the moment—to make another choice.

When I work with clients, I recommend that they ask themselves these five questions before reaching for the foods they crave. When we work on these questions together, we achieve some pretty amazing results.

1. **What's *really* happening?** Think about why you're eating when you're not hungry and the reasons you want to eat. Identify the foods you're craving and connect them to the feelings you have at that time.

2. **What do I feel?** Take inventory of your feelings. Be specific about what you are experiencing: anger, loneliness, boredom, or despair. Think about the origin of those feelings and the reasons you are focusing in that moment on what's missing from your life rather than what you actually have going for yourself.

3. **What do I need?** Could it be that you need more sleep or help with a project or direction for your goals? Maybe a babysitter or some "me time"? Take stock of your needs and prioritize them in order to prevent yourself from eating compulsively. And for the love of God, please accept help. You matter.

4. **What's in the way?** Think about the barriers to getting your needs met now. What is blocking you? How can those roadblocks be removed?

5. **What tools do I have at my disposal to help me now?** Decide what nonfood steps you can take to manage your emotional needs in the moment.

In the Next Chapter: Success with the **F-15** Plan

Once you start to understand the feelings that trigger emotional eating, you can use mindful eating and journal writing to fully explore those feelings. Then, you can practice making informed decisions about what to do in response to these feelings. When you experience cravings, you can use other foods or activities to distract yourself from the foods you crave. Or you can have just a taste of the food you desire. Practice and reflection will show you which strategies work best in different kinds of situations. These and other strategies will serve you well as you proceed to the next section of the book. Remember, the F-15 Plan is all about 15 servings, 15 pounds, and 15 days. In Chapter 3, I'll show you exactly how you can use the F-15 Plan to change your weight—and your life—for good.

Chapter 3

EATING THE F-15 WAY: 10 SUCCESS STRATEGIES THAT REALLY WORK

It's our decisions, not the conditions of our lives,
that determine our destiny.
—Tony Robbins

With the F-15 Plan, it's not just about *what* you eat, although of course that's important. Weight-loss success is much more likely if you follow some important behavioral strategies in addition to the choices you make for every meal. Based on my many years of experience working with hospital patients and the clients in my private practice, I've identified 10 Success Strategies that go a long way toward helping people stick to a weight-loss plan.

In the section that follows, I'll share my 10 Success Strategies with you, explain how and why they help, and give you tips for following them in the best possible way. These strategies are simple—no need to reorganize your life to fit them in. Just start working them into your daily routines, and before you know it, you'll be much better positioned for F-15 Success.

Success Strategy #1: Eat within the First Hour of Awakening

When you are at rest, your body wants to conserve energy, so your metabolism slows down. Just as you shut off the lights when you sleep, your body turns down many of the processes involved in metabolism. When you wake up, you want to turn everything up and start burning calories and fat as soon as possible. That's why I recommend eating breakfast within 1 hour of waking up. By eating a nutritious, energy-revving F-15 breakfast, you are jump-starting your metabolism. When you add healthy food to your tank, so to speak, you prime your engines and get them ready to go, go, go for the day, so you can do everything that you have to do as well as those things you want to do, while feeling energetic.

If you skip breakfast, you're telling your body to stay in conservation mode. You're setting yourself up to feel tired, lethargic, and irritable.

Despite what you may have heard or read, it still stands that if you skip breakfast, you're telling your body to stay in conservation mode. You're setting yourself up to feel tired, lethargic, and irritable. When no fuel comes into your tank, your body starts thinking about holding on to calories and fat rather than burning them because it doesn't know when more food will come. This is absolutely not the way you want to start your day. Even if you don't feel like having breakfast, push yourself to have something—an apple, an orange, some yogurt, maybe a glass of vegetable juice. Something is better than nothing.

And if you've heard news reports suggesting that skipping breakfast is a good way to cut calories, I'll tell you from the experiences of my clients that it always tends to backfire when they overeat during meals and snacks later on. And research backs this up: The National Weight Control Registry reports that 78 percent of successful weight losers eat breakfast every day.

What I want you to do is to change the way you think about breakfast. Enough with the heavy pancake, sausage, egg, and greasy potato meals that zap your energy by midday and weigh you down! To put more pep in your step, my latest sensation is the—wait for it—breakfast salad!

That's right; we're talking salad for breakfast. Why not? Where in the Bible does it say you can't have green vegetables for breakfast? And where in the Bible does it say that breakfast must contain some kind of fatty meat (I'm looking at you, bacon and sausage) and a pitcher of syrup or molasses? That's right—nowhere.

My favorite breakfast salad is chock-full of protein, fresh leafy greens to fight inflammation, and creamy avocado to provide just the right finish to the salty and sweet combo of red grapefruit and savory prosciutto. I'll share the recipe later in Phase 2. Breakfast salad is a time-saving phenomenon that allows you to do all of the things you have to do in your busy life. So prepare to be dazzled by this recipe. And prepare to have friends dropping over again and again once they taste it, too.

What's your excuse for skipping breakfast? Here are the most common reasons that my clients give for skipping this very important meal, along with my advice about why you shouldn't give in to it.

Excuse: "I'm not hungry in the morning." I know this happens to many people, especially women. In fact, it happens to me! I wake up and feel like I could go hours without eating. This may be due to rising levels of the stress hormone cortisol, which go down in the night and rise in the morning. It's okay not to eat the second you get out of bed. But it really is best to break your fast within an hour of waking in order to wake up your metabolism. Choose a smaller breakfast if you'd like, but don't skip it.

Excuse: "I don't have time to eat breakfast." I get it—time is short in the morning. But it's easy to throw together a healthy breakfast in seconds flat if you've made preparations the night before. For the fastest breakfast ever, add 1 tablespoon ground flaxseed or chia seeds and a dash of vanilla extract to 1 cup of low-fat Greek yogurt. Voilà! Breakfast!

Excuse: "If I skip breakfast, I'll eat fewer calories for the day." It's tempting to eliminate those early-morning calories in the quest to lose weight. But doing so doesn't actually help with weight loss; in fact, it does the opposite. Skipping breakfast puts your body in starvation mode, which slows your metabolism and impedes weight loss. And if you skip breakfast, you're likely to make up for those breakfast calories—and then some—later in the day. There is a new weight-loss strategy called intermittent fasting. This way of eating typically involves alternating daily periods of fasting. Some experts describe it as drastically cutting back on calories for short periods of time. It is based on the idea that as your body adjusts to the periods of fasting, you become more satiated by eating smaller portions and therefore consume fewer calories. Cutting portions, or rather getting your body adjusted to correct-size portions (not fasting), is the hallmark of the F-15 Plan. The difference is, you get to actually eat food, real food, and enjoy your life without starving yourself. Despite the evidence for warding off chronic diseases, such as diabetes and heart disease, I don't recommend intermittent fasting for my clients or for those of you who are on a weight-loss journey. I recommend that you start a plan you can live with for the rest of your life, not just for a short period. In my practice, I see that eating breakfast is the best way to go.

Success Strategy #2:
Eat Early and Often

Many people follow this kind of daily eating plan: They either skip breakfast or have a small bite in the morning. They go light on lunch. Then their hunger roars like a starved lion in the middle of the afternoon, at which point they start eating sweet/salty junk food. Then at dinner, thinking they didn't really eat much during the day, they help themselves to giant portions of their evening meal, followed by dessert and bowls of ice cream and chips while sitting around watching TV for a few hours before bed.

This is not the way to eat.

It's much better for your body to eat early and often. That means having a healthy, lean, green F-15 breakfast; a morning snack to keep your metabolism humming; a healthy lunch; an afternoon snack; and a dinner that's smaller than you're probably used to, with a small snack in the evening. Ideally you should eat the bulk of your calories at breakfast and lunch. Researchers have found that people who consume most of their calories before 3 p.m. are more likely to be successful at weight loss than those who pile on the calories later in the day. And get this: It takes 24 hours for your blood sugar to stabilize after a late-night meal. Eating earlier gives your body plenty of time to burn up calories and stabilize your blood sugar before you get into bed. Don't worry—you don't have to think too much about this. Just follow my F-15 Plan and you'll get exactly what you need, when you need it.

Success Strategy #3:
Get 7 to 8 Hours of Sleep per Night

We Americans are an exhausted bunch of people. Although sleep researchers recommend 7 to 8 hours per night, studies show that

30 percent of us get fewer than 6 hours of sleep a night. Being chronically tired truly interferes with your health. Lack of sleep is associated with higher rates of hypertension, diabetes, depression, obesity, and cancer. In fact, studies show that getting fewer than 5 hours of sleep per night is associated with a higher body-mass index. The more sleep-deprived you are, the higher your risk of obesity. Insomnia causes hormonal changes and cravings for carbohydrates. And when you deprive yourself of adequate sleep, fatigue lowers your ability to resist trigger foods. Instead of eating, try taking a power nap for a bigger, more effective payoff.

Nighttime sleep even has an effect on daytime hunger, influencing the production of the hormones that regulate appetite. When we're overtired, we tend to eat more than we do when we are well rested. Overall, people who sleep less appear to weigh more. Be sure to get your 7 to 8 hours a night. If you're having trouble sleeping, see your doctor; you may have a sleep disorder, such as sleep apnea. If you have trouble getting the sleep you need, try these fabulous sleep boosters.

Avoid stimulants near bedtime. Caffeine, alcohol, and nicotine too close to bedtime can rev you up and rob you of sleep. As we get older, caffeine can affect us more, so even if you used to be able to sleep like a baby despite late-in-the day coffee consumption, don't be surprised if you notice that your tolerance is going down. Alcohol before bed can interrupt sleep, as well. As for nicotine, you'll be healthier in so many ways if you quit smoking altogether.

Stick to a schedule. Try to go to bed and get up at the same time each day. Sleep no longer than an hour later on days off.

Exercise—but not too late in the day. Daytime exercise can improve your sleep, but don't schedule your workouts too close to bedtime because they may keep you awake. The effect of exercise on sleep varies from person to person, but if you're having trouble catching your zzz's, try doing your workout earlier in the day.

Don't eat before bed. I'll tell you more about this soon, but for now, know that restful sleep is most likely to occur if you stop eating at least 3 hours before bedtime.

Create a sleep-friendly bedroom. In general, we sleep best in a room that is cool, dark, and quiet. Use shades, earplugs, fans, white-noise machines, eyeshades, and whatever else you need to make your bedroom conducive to successful sleep.

Follow a relaxing bedtime routine. Meditate, take a warm bath, listen to soothing music (I find that a good orgasm always helps, too!). Do whatever relaxes you for 15 minutes or so before you go to sleep.

Keep electronics out of the bedroom. Some studies have found that the light emitted from cell phones, laptops, televisions, and e-readers can keep us awake. Avoid using them in the bedroom or before you go to sleep.

Check in with your doctor. If you're having trouble going to sleep, staying asleep, or waking up in the morning, tell your doctor. Millions of Americans have sleep disorders, and some medications list sleep problems as a side effect. Your doctor can help diagnose the causes of sleep problems and can educate you about treatment options. One of these sleep problems is sleep apnea, and I have a very personal reason for telling you to take this sleep disorder very seriously.

First, let me tell you a little about sleep apnea. It is a surprisingly common condition in which a person's breathing pauses or becomes very shallow during sleep. Breathing pauses can last for a few seconds or even a minute or longer and may occur as often as 30 times per hour. Having sleep apnea disrupts your sleep and can cause excessive daytime sleepiness. It can also raise your risk of high blood pressure, heart attack, stroke, obesity, and diabetes, as well as traffic accidents.

Sleep apnea is more likely to occur in people who are overweight or obese. Fat in the neck can interfere with the passage of air through the windpipe. Signs of sleep apnea include: headaches in the morning; problems with memory, concentration, or learning; irritability, depression, mood swings, or changes in personality; frequent awakening during the night to urinate; and waking up with a sore throat or dry mouth.

Sleep apnea often goes undiagnosed, and many people who have it don't realize it unless a sleep partner or family member notices loud snoring, gasping during sleep, or unusual breathing patterns. I noticed it in my husband. He is a snorer, which I've grown accustomed to, but this particular night I noticed a snoring sound different from any other I'd heard before, coupled with long pauses of no breathing, which scared the bejesus out of me! He also had begun falling asleep in the middle of conversations. At first I thought he was tired because as an emergency medicine physician he worked long hours, often at night during the third shift. That meant he worked as most people slept. So I asked him to do a sleep study, where his breathing patterns and oxygen levels were monitored and analyzed while he slept in a testing facility. The diagnosis was sleep apnea. What we discovered was that his oxygen level would drop to a dangerous low, putting him at risk for a preventable early death.

I cannot tell you how important it is to have a loved one evaluated if you even think he or she could be at risk. In my case, the neurologist who evaluated my husband believed I might have saved his life. But in the case of my cousin, who also had sleep apnea and heart disease, we weren't as fortunate.

Because of my personal stories, I beg of you: If you think you or a loved one could have sleep apnea, or if either of you has any signs of the condition, please see your doctor. Sleep apnea can be treated by sleeping with a breathing device called a CPAP (continuous positive airway pressure) machine, and treatment could also include losing weight, avoiding alcohol, changing sleep positions, and quitting smoking, as well as mouthpieces or surgery.

Success Strategy #4:
Eat Snacks That Are No Larger
Than Your Closed Fist

Incorporating snacks into your daily meal plan is a helpful way to prevent hunger and to stick to the F-15 program. But in order to stay on track, you have to make sure your snacks are a reasonable size. One of the easiest ways to do this is to eat snacks that are no larger than your closed fist. The exception to this is free foods (leafy green vegetables, which contribute few calories) and calorie-free beverages, such as coffee and tea. For example, a closed fist holds about half an ounce (1 tablespoon) of nuts. But remember, I'm talking about a *closed* fist, not an open palm.

We'll talk more about the best foods for snacking and the most effective way to schedule snacks when we delve into the details of each phase of the F-15 Plan.

Success Strategy #5:
Drink Half Your Body Weight in Water

Drinking water helps fill your stomach and boosts your body's metabolism. It also keeps you hydrated, which is important because often we mistake thirst for hunger, leading us to eat high-calorie snacks when all our bodies really want is a glass of water. To figure out how much water to drink, divide your weight in half. If you're 160 pounds, aim for about 80 ounces (10 8-ounce glasses) per day. Liquids such as unsweetened coffee, tea, and seltzer can also count in your daily tally.

But keep in mind that caffeinated beverages, though acceptable, are also diuretics, meaning the caffeine dehydrates your body and makes you pee. A good way to offset this effect is to drink a glass of water for each cup of coffee or tea you consume. Make the water ice cold, because drinking cold water revs up the metabolism even more. Your body has to work harder to stabilize its temperature and, in so doing, burns more calories for you. Winner!

To add pizazz to water and seltzer, make grape-cubes. Place a grape or two in each section of an ice cube tray, and then fill with water. Once they're frozen, pop these grape-cubes into water for a refreshing, tasty drink. This works for cut pieces of almost any of your favorite fruits. Think pineapple, mango, berries, peaches, nectarines, and melon.

Success Strategy #6: Cut Out Soda and Sugary Drinks

I can't emphasize enough how incredibly important this is. According to an *Ad Age* magazine report, Americans drank 44.7 gallons of carbonated soft drinks, 11.5 gallons of sports beverages, and 10.3 gallons of tea per person, per year. It is no secret that Americans consume more sugary soda, sweetened iced tea, and other high-sugar beverages than water, daily. According to the Centers for Disease Control and Prevention, sugary drink consumption is associated with obesity, diabetes, heart disease, and other health problems. Here's why this is important to you. Your weight loss is at stake, and nixing sugary beverages from your diet can be a huge boon to your success. By eliminating sugary beverages, the average American could lose about 15 pounds in a year without making any other changes. And that's just the average American who drinks the equivalent of about one can of soda per day (I know plenty of people who drink three, four, or five cans—or more—every day).

Do yourself a favor and stop drinking liquid sugar. And remember, this includes sweet tea (whadup, Alabama and Georgia!), which is loaded with sugar and calories. Try making your iced tea without sugar, flavoring it with fresh mint, ginger, or a splash of lemon, lime, orange, peach, mango, even cucumber, instead (the citrus and cucumber are alkaline in nature and reduce inflammation in the body). It may take some getting used to, but before you know it, you'll love it—and when you take a sip of sweet tea, you'll wonder how you could stand that overly sweet taste!

Numerous studies link the consumption of sweetened beverages with higher rates of diabetes and obesity. No surprise there. It makes perfect sense that if sugary drinks lead to weight gain, they'll lead to a higher risk of diabetes, since the two are linked. But here's a finding that suggests sugary drinks in and of themselves influence the development of diabetes. A 2015 study published in the *BMJ* found that drinking sugar-sweetened beverages boosts diabetes risk, even among slender people and in small amounts. According to the study, compared with people who drink no sugary soft drinks, normal-weight people who consume one sweet drink a day have a 13 percent higher risk of developing diabetes.

Switching to diet sodas may not be the solution, even though they contain many fewer calories than sugar-sweetened drinks. The same study, as well as others, found that people who drink diet sodas have a higher risk of diabetes than those who don't. This is referred to as the diet-soda paradox. Although researchers don't fully understand why drinking diet soda wouldn't lower diabetes risk, they believe it may be that artificial sweeteners encourage sugar cravings and dependence and that their sweet taste enhances human appetite even though they provide no calories.

It surely does make sense to me. On *The Dr. Oz Show*, we tested a small sample of audience members, comparing those who regularly consumed artificial sweeteners with those who did not. Each was given the choice of a slice of cake or a larger hunk of cake. The people who regularly consumed artificial sweeteners chose the hunk of cake because their cravings and preferences for sweet foods had increased with their consumption of artificial sweeteners, which are sometimes more than 10 times sweeter than sugar itself. The routine use of artificial sweeteners,

The routine use of artificial sweeteners, one Harvard study says, can even change the way you taste healthy foods, like fruits and vegetables.

one Harvard study says, can even change the way you taste healthy foods, like fruits and vegetables. Researchers say the intensity of sweetness in zero-calorie sweeteners can retrain your brain, making healthy, high-fiber produce taste unappealing and possibly preventing you from associating sweetness with calorie intake. The result, you wonder? You crave more sweets, tend to choose sweet foods over nutritious alternatives, and ultimately gain weight. Boom!

Success Strategy #7:
Avoid Eating within
3 Hours of Going to Bed

At the end of the day, your digestive system needs to slow down and rest, so I recommend that you avoid eating anything within 3 hours of bedtime. Eating before bed can interfere with sleep quality and throw off your circadian rhythms. It can also contribute to heartburn and acid reflux. If you must eat before bed, choose a small protein-rich snack, such as a cup of yogurt.

Success Strategy #8:
Use a Daily Food Diary

Keeping track of everything you eat and drink can truly help with weight loss. I've seen it among the people I've worked with, and research backs it up, as well. In fact, one large study found that keeping a food diary can actually double your weight loss. That's right—the simple act of writing down what you eat can dramatically increase your chances of success. You've got to love the fact that something so easy has the potential to do so much!

Why does writing in a food diary make a difference? There are a few reasons. One is that tracking your food makes you think more about the foods that you choose to eat. Mindless eating is one of the biggest contributors to weight gain, and keeping a food diary helps to get your mind back into the correct process of eating. Reflecting on what you eat, when you eat it, and the emotions you feel before, during, and after eating can help you to understand the habits and emotions that impact your eating choices.

Looking back at your food diary gives you an opportunity to identify trends and unconscious habits—for example, you may realize that you overeat on days that you work late or that you do a fantastic job of sticking to your eating goals on days that you exercise vigorously. These kinds of patterns are different for each one of us, and one of the best ways to understand your own individual patterns is to put everything in writing.

Using a food diary also helps to up your accountability—to yourself. By writing down everything you eat, including the "cheat foods," you give yourself space to be honest with yourself, which is one of the first steps toward true mindfulness. With accountability and honesty comes true acknowledgment of what you're doing, how it's helping or harming you, and what you can do to improve your habits and your health.

You can use any kind of food diary you like—paper or electronic. Some of my clients prefer a spiral notebook; others choose one of those fancy leather journals. And many are drawn to online programs and smartphone apps that make it easy to track food and fitness activities. It doesn't matter what you use as long as you keep on top of what you're eating and, if relevant, the reasons you eat what you choose to in the moment.

Success Strategy #9: Shop with a List

Always use a shopping list when you go to the grocery store; it is a sure-fire way to cut back on junk food. Not only will this save you from eating food you hadn't planned on eating, but it will help you to lose weight and save you money, too. By sticking to the foods on your list and refusing to buy other, unplanned foods, you spend the money that you previously planned to spend, which supports your calorie and weekly or monthly food budget, as well. Using a grocery list is an example of what's referred to as a precommitment strategy. These kinds of strategies help build momentum for success because they allow your present and future selves to work together. When you write a grocery list, your

(continued on page 50)

My **F-15** *Food Diary*

DATE	DAY OF THE WEEK	MEAL PLAN PHASE WEEK & DAY

	BREAKFAST	MORNING SNACK	LUNCH
Time			
# Ounces of Water			
# Protein Servings			
# Vegetable Servings			
# Fruit Servings			
# Dairy Servings			
# Fat Servings			
#Grain Servings			
My Feelings and Emotions Before and/or After Eating			

☑ Daily multivitamin   ☑ Daily probiotic supplement

AFTERNOON SNACK	DINNER	EVENING SNACK	TOTAL SERVINGS FOR DAY

present self is promising your future self that you will make smart choices in the grocery store. This commitment can spread out to other choices, as well.

In a study published in the journal *Nutrition & Diabetes*, Australian researchers found that women who used shopping lists lost an average of 27 pounds (9 more pounds than those who did not use lists). Ultimately, these researchers found that planning your meals ahead of time by creating shopping lists helps you to gauge food intake better and stick to the meal plan while avoiding the pitfalls of strategically placed, unplanned treats that you might otherwise buy on impulse at the grocery store. Their results support the reasons that I have used shopping lists for my entire career to help clients stick not only to their food budget but to their calorie budget, as well!

To make it easier for you to create useful grocery lists, I've included lists of recommended foods to buy in each phase of the F-15 Plan. That should make life easier for you!

Success Strategy #10:
Take Special Care If You Work Nights

Many people work overnight shifts. According to the Bureau of Labor Statistics, almost 15 million Americans work full-time on evening shifts, night shifts, rotating shifts, or other irregular schedules. Unfortunately, shift work can make it harder to lose weight. But by taking steps to accommodate your erratic schedule, you can slim down successfully using the F-15 Plan.

Shift work disrupts your circadian rhythms, which are the physical, mental, and behavioral changes that follow a 24-hour cycle (think of it as a clock) within your body. Circadian rhythms are directed by environmental cues such as sunlight, darkness, and temperature. People who work night shifts often experience disruption of their circadian rhythms, which affects their sleeping and eating patterns. Because of circadian rhythm disorders, people who do shift work can have higher rates of heart disease and mental health conditions such as depression. Shift workers are also more likely than 9-5 workers to be overweight or obese.

Maintaining a healthy weight is a bit harder for shift workers for several reasons. Shift working requires you to sleep during the day and work during the night, forcing you to go against your body's natural rhythm. As a result, your metabolism can slow down, which reduces your body's calorie and fat burning potential. Shift workers may also eat more because their mealtimes get mixed up. And if they don't get enough sleep, exhaustion may negatively impact the action of their hunger and satiety hormones. It can also be more difficult for shift workers to get the exercise they need, and it may be harder for them to schedule stress-relief techniques into their daily life. If you're a shift worker, you can optimize your weight-loss success by taking these steps.

Follow the F-15 Plan closely. It's tempting to snack on sweets, chips, and other junk food, especially when you're up in the middle of the night working while most of the rest of the world is fast asleep. Try really hard to resist those temptations and to stick with F-15 meals and snacks. Pack meals and snacks at home, and take them to work in a cooler so you're not a prisoner of your environment, getting stuck trying to make healthy meals out of vending machine fare.

Schedule your meals. Eat breakfast within an hour of waking and eat dinner at least 3 hours before bed. An overnight worker may have breakfast at 2 p.m., lunch at 7 p.m., and dinner at 2 a.m., with snacks spread out in-between. Figure out the meal schedule that works best for you and stick to it every day, even if you're not working. And resist the urge to grab a big greasy breakfast after work! Not only will it pile on hundreds of excess calories, but it will also interfere with your sleep and slow down your metabolism.

Schedule your sleep. Do your best to get 7 to 8 hours of sleep at the same time every day. This can help minimize the impact of circadian rhythm disorder. Experts recommend sleeping during the day even on your days off in order to stick to a sleep schedule. This can be hard, because you end up missing social events and other things that go on during the day. But do your best to sleep at the same time each day and to get enough sleep, which is key.

Make a plan for exercise. The good news is that gyms tend to be less crowded during the day, when you're home from work. Try to exercise at about the same time each day, and for your best chance of serene, deep sleep, get the workout in at least a couple of hours before bed. Remember, exercise raises endorphin levels so it's likely that a workout will pump you up, interfering with a restful sleep experience.

Schedule relaxation. Whether you enjoy meditating, doing yoga, or engaging in other relaxation techniques, be sure to fit some kind of relaxation into each day.

Seek help if you need it. If you are having trouble sleeping or dealing with mood swings or have any other health problems related to your shift work, by all means, please see your doctor.

F-15 Serving Sizes

Choosing the right foods is an important part of the F-15 Plan. But there's more to smart eating than making optimal food choices. Making sure that you eat the right *amount* of food is crucial, too. Even when we choose the healthiest foods, our serving sizes tend to be way too big.

There's a very good reason for this. Portion sizes in restaurants have grown like crazy over the past few decades. If you want to see this in action, go for a meal at Olive Garden, Applebee's, Cheesecake Factory, or just about any other family-style restaurant chain. Check out the sizes of the appetizers, soups, entrées, desserts—even the salads and other "healthy" fare. The serving sizes are sometimes two or three times larger than the serving sizes many of us grew up with, and they're much larger than those we should be eating. Many of the selections at these restaurant chains can be more than 1,000 calories per serving. Some are a whopping 1,500 calories or more!

What concerns me is that these oversize restaurant portions have trained our eyes to see normal, healthy-size portions as being way too small. What we now think of as normal is much more food than our bodies require for nutritional support. When you're accustomed to getting burritos as big as your forearm at Chipotle or Boloco or believing that a 32-ounce soft drink at any fast-food restaurant is a normal serving size, then you start thinking that way at home, too. Once that happens, it's hard to trust yourself to eyeball healthy serving sizes, because when you do, you dish out two, three, or four times more than you ought to be eating—not only for the body that you want, but also for the body that you currently have now. You're being set up by the restaurant industry, who may be aiming to give you value for your dollar, but in the end you pay again with your body. Ahhh, but there's help for you. Keep reading and you'll see that I've got you covered.

The need to master and navigate proper portion sizes isn't restricted to just soft drinks and restaurant foods. I need you to understand how to portion out healthy food, too. Take cashews and almonds, for example. These are superhealthy foods. But if you eat too many of them, you're setting yourself up for weight gain. Snack on a handful, not half a tub, of them. The same is true with avocados—again, a mega healthy food. But a serving is not an entire avocado; it's a quarter. And vegetables—go ahead and eat as much roasted cauliflower as you want, provided it's not glistening with oil. Even the healthiest foods lead to weight gain if they're eaten in supersize portions.

Don't feel bad if your serving-estimation skills are off-kilter. Studies have found that even card-carrying, credentialed nutrition experts trained in the field have trouble estimating portion sizes. The gigantic serving sizes in restaurants have muddied the waters for all of us.

For this reason, one of the most important things to keep top of mind in this plan is portion sizes. In this section, I'll show you what healthy portion sizes *really* are. I'll give you charts that show you how much of each food is a healthy portion size. But don't worry: I'm not going to ask you to keep measuring spoons in your pocket or a food scale in your purse. Instead, I'll share with you a few very simple visual guides that will retrain your eyes so you'll be able to estimate serving sizes without having to play around with all kinds of measuring tools. If you like to measure and weigh, that's fine; but I want this to be easy, so I'll show you how to eyeball foods accurately.

Once you've mastered the art of estimating portion sizes, we'll move on to the heart and soul of the F-15 Plan, and I'll show you how to lose weight simply and easily by eating 15 servings of delicious, healthy foods every day. Let's start with vegetables since they are some of the most nutritious, most filling foods on the table.

VEGETABLES

Vegetable Serving Sizes

FOOD	SERVING SIZE
Cooked vegetables	½ cup—about the size of a tennis ball
Vegetable juice	½ cup
Raw vegetables, chopped	1 cup—the size of a man's closed fist
Leafy greens, such as lettuce or spinach	2 cups—the size of two men's closed fists

Tips for Choosing Vegetables

Vegetables provide a huge amount of nutritional support. And making them a big part of your diet can deliver so many health benefits. Not only do they fill you up and help to sustain and prepare your body for its normal functions, but they provide vitamins, minerals, antioxidants, and phytochemicals that actually help to lower your risk of diseases such as heart disease, diabetes, hypertension, and certain forms of cancer.

And if that's not enough reason for you to eat more veggies, consider the fact that they will aid in your weight loss. Vegetables are naturally lower in calories than most other foods, and although nutrient-rich, they are also high-volume, which means they contain lots of water. This is a big reason for you to eat more of them, because they will help you to lose water weight. The more water you put into your body, the more you lose. Now I ask you, what's not to love about that? As you plan your daily veggie intake, keep the following tips in mind.

Select a rainbow of colors. The pigments in vegetables contain various antioxidants, which are substances that fight free radicals that cause damage in your body's cells. Antioxidants act as a built-in repair system, protecting your body against premature aging and disease. Plant-based antioxidants include vitamins A, C, and E, as well as alpha-carotene, beta-carotene, lutein, lycopene, and zeaxanthin. To get a full range of these amazing nutrients, choose dark green, red, yellow, purple, and orange vegetables. You don't have to eat all of the various colors every day, but try to include some from each color group throughout the week.

Buy vegetables in season. Fresh, in-season vegetables are tastiest and are often lower in price than they are when bought off-season. Frozen vegetables are just as nutritious and an economical alternative.

Buy and freeze. When vegetables are on sale or in season, buy extra and freeze what you can't eat.

Try new vegetables on a regular basis. Like most people, you probably see vegetables in the produce aisle that you have no idea how to cook or eat. Make it an exciting project to try new veggies every week or every month. Look online or in cookbooks for preparation ideas and educate yourself about ways to incorporate new vegetables into your diet.

Focus on convenience. The easier it is to eat vegetables, the more likely you are to include them in meals and snacks. If your budget allows it, buy precut vegetables. Or spend a few minutes a day washing, peeling, and cutting up vegetables for the next day's meals. And don't forget frozen vegetables, which are as nutritious as fresh. Just be sure to select "naked" varieties without butter, seasonings, or sauces. Canned vegetables are fine if they're naked; choose brands without added salt or seasonings, or rinse canned vegetables before cooking.

Jump off the iceberg. We're all so accustomed to eating iceberg lettuce in salads and sandwiches. But the truth is, iceberg lettuce has hardly any nutrients at all. The darker the green in leafy green vegetables, the more nutritious they are. Try adding different kinds of lettuces to your salads, such as romaine, butterhead, and leaf lettuces, as well as greens, like spinach, lacinato and baby kale, arugula, and watercress. To wean yourself off of iceberg, start by mixing in small amounts of these other lettuces and greens to your salads, increasing the ratio over time. If you're like many of my clients, once you become accustomed to the bold, spicy taste of these other leafy salad choices, you'll never go back to boring old iceberg lettuce again.

Tuck veggies into other foods. Take a lesson from parents who try to sneak vegetables into the tummies of their fussy-eater kids. You can sneak vegetables into all kinds of foods, including soups, smoothies, stews, dips, casseroles, pies, pizza, stir-fries, and sauces.

Invite vegetables to your breakfast table. We're used to relegating veggies to lunch and dinner, but there's no reason not to include them in your breakfast, as well. Add them to smoothies or omelets or breakfast bowls, as you'll see in your F-15 meal plan, or just crunch on them in the raw. And make sure to try my veggie-rich breakfast recipes, such as breakfast salads and veggie-egg scrambles.

Don't confuse vegetables with "veggie snacks." Many of these snacks boasting green beans, spinach, and other real vegetables may not contain vegetables at all! Instead, they are nothing more than dressed up junk food masquerading as healthy options, often made with vegetable powder and mostly processed wheat flour or that of another grain. So just because a snack food says it "contains vegetables" doesn't mean it's good for you or that it belongs in your daily meal plan. Read the fine print: The chips that say they contain sweet potatoes, broccoli, or any other veggie usually also contain lots of fat, calories, salt, and sometimes even sugar. They're also not very satiating, so you'll still feel hungry after you gobble them up.

Leave these products on the shelf and stick with fresh produce items. They're better for you, much more filling, and far more likely to help you achieve your weight-loss goals. If you enjoy them as chips, as I do, toss thinly sliced versions of your favorites in extra virgin olive oil, add a pinch of sea salt, and roast or bake at 350°F for a few minutes.

Everyday Vegetables and Occasional Vegetables

Certain vegetables are low enough in calories that I recommend eating four to six servings a day (depending on which F-15 phase you're in). I refer to these as Everyday Vegetables. However, a small number of vegetables are high enough in calories and carbohydrates that I recommend not going overboard with them. These vegetables, which I refer to as Occasional Vegetables, are not included in Phase 1 of the F-15 Plan. During Phase 2 and Phase 3, go ahead and enjoy up to two servings a week.

Everyday Vegetables include:

Arugula	Endive	Radishes
Asparagus	Escarole	Rutabaga
Bean sprouts, broccoli sprouts, alfalfa sprouts	Green beans	Spaghetti squash
	Jicama	Spinach
	Kale	Sugar snap peas
Beets	Leeks	Summer squash (zucchini)
Bell peppers	Lettuces (artisan, leaf, curly green, romaine, butterhead)	Swiss chard
Broccoli		Tomatoes
Brussels sprouts		Turnip greens
Cabbage	Mushrooms	Turnips
Cauliflower	Mustard greens	Water chestnuts
Celery	Okra	Watercress
Chicory	Onions	Wax beans
Collard greens	Parsnips	
Cucumber	Radicchio	

Occasional Vegetables. Eat these only in Phase 2 and Phase 3 of the F-15 Plan. You get to have two servings a week that count as part of your F-15 daily serving tally. Occasional vegetables include:

Acorn squash	Green peas	Pumpkin
Butternut squash	Plantain	Sweet potatoes
Carrots	Potatoes	or yams
Corn		

FRUITS

Fruit Serving Sizes

FOOD	SERVING SIZE
Whole fruit (apples, bananas, citrus fruit, mango, peaches, pears, etc.)	½ large or 1 small—about the size of a baseball
Berries, cherries, grapes, melon, pineapple, papaya, or other small or chopped fruit	½ cup—about the size of a lightbulb
Dried fruit	¼ cup—about the diameter of a golf ball
Fruit juice	½ cup—about half the size of a small milk carton

Tips for Choosing Fruits

Like vegetables, fruits contain a cornucopia of nutrients, including vitamins, minerals, and antioxidants. As you plan your daily menus, keep these tips in mind.

Select a rainbow of colors. As with vegetables, selecting a range of different color fruits provides you with a variety of nutrients. Mix it up, including blue, red, orange, and yellow fruits throughout your week.

Choose different kinds of fruits. Berries bring different health benefits to the table than citrus fruits; the same is true for melons, stone fruit, and other types of fruit. To make sure you get all of the benefits that fruit has to offer, help yourself to some of each.

Bring on the berries. Thanks to their superhigh levels of antioxidants, berries—blueberries, strawberries, raspberries, and blackberries—should be frequent guests on your table. Studies have found that berries offer a host of nutritional benefits, reducing the risk of everything from heart disease, high blood pressure, and diabetes to some kinds of cancer and even cognitive decline. Eat them fresh, blend them into smoothies, plop them into yogurt, or eat them right from the freezer. Speaking of smoothies, here's a great tip: Instead of making just one smoothie, multiply the recipe and make two, four, six, or more servings. Pour what's leftover into single-serving containers and stick them in the freezer. Then when you're ready to have one, toss it into the blender and give it a spin. Note: This works best for smoothies that contain no yogurt. For those with yogurt, leave the yogurt out when you make your big batch. Then mix in the yogurt just before you're ready to have your smoothie.

Buy fruits in season. Fresh, in-season fruits are incredibly delicious. Is there anything more wonderful than a strawberry right off the vine, an apple fresh from the orchard, or a peach straight from the farm? I don't think so. Stock up on these delectable fruits while they're in season. Cut up and freeze whatever you can't eat. And by all means, shop at your local farmers' markets, co-ops, and street vendors who bring fresh produce from the farm to your community.

Rely on frozen fruit. Frozen berries, mango chunks, and other fruit often tastes better than out-of-season fresh fruit. And frozen fruit is superconvenient for smoothies. Even canned fruit is okay if it's packed in its own juice. Make sure to choose "naked" fruit without any sugar or sweetened syrups. Keep bananas on hand in the freezer for desserts, smoothies, and protein bars.

Focus on convenience. Spend a few minutes a day washing, peeling, and cutting up fruit for the next day's meals. If your wallet allows, buy precut fruit in your grocery store's produce aisle.

A RAINBOW OF CHOICES

You can make sure you get all of the amazing nutrients from all of the different colors of produce by including these multihued fruits and veggies in your weekly eating plan.

Red: Tomatoes, red bell peppers, beets, strawberries, watermelon

Blue/Purple: Blackberries, eggplant, radicchio, raisins, grapes, blueberries, blue potatoes (which are really purple in color), purple carrots, plums, purple cabbage

Green: Collard greens, broccoli, turnip greens, Brussels sprouts, green beans, asparagus, lacinato and baby kale

Orange: Pumpkin, mango, sweet potato, apricots, peaches, butternut squash, oranges, orange bell peppers, carrots

Yellow: Summer squash, yellow bell peppers, pineapple, lemon, guava, bananas

GOING ORGANIC

Q: **Should I buy organic produce? Is it worth the higher price?**

A: Organic fruits and vegetables do cost more than conventionally grown produce. But I think that for some kinds of fruits and vegetables, organic is worth the extra money. I go with the advice of the Environmental Working Group (EWG), an organization that measures the pesticide residue found on produce in the United States. Each year, EWG comes up with two lists: the "Dirty Dozen," which includes the produce items with the most pesticide residue, and the "Clean 15," which have the least. I recommend buying organic when you're choosing Dirty Dozen produce. Sticking with standard is fine with the Clean 15. (To learn more about EWG's work, visit EWG.org.) Here are the most current lists.

✓ **The Dirty Dozen:** Apples, peaches, nectarines, strawberries, grapes, celery, spinach, bell peppers, cucumbers, cherry tomatoes, imported snap peas, and potatoes

✓ **The Clean 15:** Avocado, sweet corn, pineapple, cabbage, frozen sweet peas, onions, asparagus, mango, papaya, kiwifruit, eggplant, grapefruit, cantaloupe, cauliflower, and sweet potatoes

DAIRY

Dairy Serving Sizes

FOOD	SERVING SIZE
Milk (low-fat)	1 cup
Yogurt (low-fat)	1 cup (8-ounce container) or 5.3 ounces of Greek yogurt
Hard cheese (low-fat), such as cheddar, mozzarella, Swiss, Parmesan	1 ounce—about the size of a domino
Soft cheese (ricotta, cottage, queso fresco, queso blanco, etc.)	½ cup
Milk alternatives: Soy milk and unsweetened nut milks (low-fat and calcium-fortified when possible)	1 cup

Tips for Choosing Dairy Foods

Dairy foods provide some very important nutrients. The calcium and vitamin D in dairy foods help your body build and maintain bone mass, which is especially important for women because it may reduce the risk of osteoporosis. The potassium in dairy foods can positively impact your blood pressure; in fact, intake of low-fat dairy products is associated with a reduced risk of high blood pressure, cardiovascular disease, and diabetes. Here are some tips on making the smartest choices when including dairy foods in your meal plan.

Select low-fat dairy foods. Because of their high fat content, full-fat dairy foods contain many more calories than low-fat varieties. So choose low-fat dairy instead. Occasional fat-free dairy foods are acceptable, but bear in mind that we need some fat to help absorb fat-soluble vitamins.

Buy unsweetened yogurt. Flavored yogurts can contain as much added sugar as candy; in fact, some brands actually come with candy mix-ins! Stay away from yogurt flavored with sugary fruits, vanilla, high-fat granolas, and other ingredients. Choose low-fat unflavored yogurt, either regular or Greek. I prefer Greek yogurt because it is higher in protein and lower in carbohydrates.

Make smart substitutions. If you have trouble digesting dairy because of lactose intolerance, choose lactose-free products. You may be okay with yogurt, which sometimes doesn't bother lactose-intolerant people. If you choose not to eat animal products, opt for low-fat soy or nut milks instead of cow's milk, and pick a brand that is fortified with calcium. I'm not crazy about soy cheeses because of the amount of processing they undergo, but if you must eat soy cheese, select low-fat varieties. If you don't consume dairy, you can still get the calcium your body needs. Here's how: Drink calcium-fortified soy milk, fruit juice, or nut milk; choose calcium-fortified soy products, such as tofu; eat canned fish with bones, such as sardines and salmon; and eat calcium-rich greens, such as collards, turnip greens, kale, and bok choy. Another option is to take calcium supplements of 1,000 to 1,500 milligrams daily. If you do take calcium supplements, have them with a protein-rich meal, since protein helps your body make the best use of calcium.

Understand what you're getting with nut milks. Many people substitute nut milk for dairy milk, but it's really not an even swap. Nut milk doesn't provide the protein that dairy milk or nuts have. For example, 1 cup of almond or coconut milk contains 1 gram of protein compared to 8 grams of protein found in 1 cup of cow's milk. Basically, the nutrient composition does not match that of cow's milk, but nut milk can be a substitute for flavor and texture. If you do choose to drink nut milks as a substitute for animal milk, select unsweetened varieties fortified with calcium and make up for the protein with other protein-rich foods.

PROTEINS

Protein Serving Sizes

FOOD	SERVING SIZE
Meat (lean beef, pork, ham) and poultry (chicken or turkey without skin)	3–4 ounces—about the size of a deck of cards or the palm of your hand, minus your fingers
Canadian bacon	3–4 slices
Turkey, beef, or pork bacon	2 slices
Fatty fish (salmon, tuna, sardines, mackerel, trout)	3–4 ounces—the size of a checkbook
Canned water-packed tuna	3 ounces
White fish (cod, scrod, tilapia, grouper, bass, haddock, catfish, snapper, etc.)	4 ounces—the size of a checkbook
Shellfish (clams, oysters, shrimp, scallops, etc.)	4 ounces
Eggs	1 egg or 3 egg whites
Nuts (peanuts, almonds, pistachios, walnuts, pecans, etc.); note that nuts are also listed under Fats and Oils	1 ounce
Nut butters (peanut, pecan, almond, etc.); note that nut butters are also listed under Fats and Oils	2 tablespoons—about the size of a poker chip
Seeds (pumpkin, sunflower, chia, flax, etc.)	1 ounce
Cooked beans (black, kidney, pinto, white), peas (chickpeas, cowpeas, split peas), and lentils	½ cup
Soy (tofu, tempeh, roasted soybeans, edamame)	½ cup
Hummus	4 tablespoons

Tips for Choosing Proteins

Protein is one of the most important macronutrients in the F-15 Plan. High-protein foods—such as meat, poultry, fish, beans, nuts, and seeds—contain a variety of nutrients, including B vitamins (niacin, thiamin, riboflavin, and B$_6$), vitamin E, iron, zinc, and magnesium. They help build strong muscles, bones, blood, skin, and cartilage, as well as hormones and enzymes. They also help with weight loss. Keep these suggestions in mind as you pick your F-15 Plan proteins.

Make it lean. Choose the leanest cuts of beef (eye of round, fillet, sirloin, top round) and cut off all visible fat. Choose white-meat poultry, and remove all skin and fat.

Cook it lean. Choose cooking methods that require little or no added fat, such as baking, broiling, and grilling. If you do use fat, be sure to choose from your F-15 Plan fat allowances.

Limit red meat. Red meat is one of those foods that has both pros and cons. In its favor is the fact that red meat contains many essential nutrients, including protein, vitamin B$_6$, vitamin B$_{12}$, and iron. But there are reasons to limit it, too. Red meat intake has been associated with an increase in heart disease, colorectal cancer, and diabetes risk. For these reasons, I recommend limiting red meat to no more than three times a week. When affordable, buy grass-fed and organic grass-fed red meats, which are leaner and have a greater nutritional content.

Make fish and shellfish part of your plan. Certain kinds of seafood—such as salmon, trout, sardines, herring, anchovies, and mackerel—are wonderful sources of omega-3 fatty acids, which are linked to a lower risk of heart disease, rheumatoid arthritis, and depression. Eat at least two or three servings a week.

Choose fresh rather than processed meats. Processed meats—ham, sausage, hot dogs, and deli meats—not only contain high amounts of sodium and (often) fat but also have been shown to raise the risk of cancer. Choose fresh meats instead.

Shake off the salt. We eat too much salt (sodium). Excessive salt can contribute to high blood pressure and heart disease. Choose meats without added sodium and nuts without salt.

Use soy sparingly. Soy milk, tofu, and edamame are fine. But I don't recommend manufactured soy food products, such as soy protein powder and other meat analogs, whose nutritional value is inferior to the real food. If you want protein, you're better off choosing nuts, seeds, or legumes as plant-based options. And if you must add an extra boost of protein to your smoothies or shakes, choose hemp protein (vegan); almond, peanut, or other nut butters; peanut powder; or low-fat milk.

All of these examples are superior to manufactured isolated soy products. Although not a plant option, whey protein concentrate (dairy) can be an acceptable backup to the real thing in a pinch.

Eat the best meat, poultry, and fish you can afford. When you walk through the protein aisle in your grocery store or butcher shop, deciding what kind of meat, poultry, and fish to buy can be a real challenge. There's organic, grass-fed, free-range, conventionally grown, farmed, hormone-free—the list is practically endless. Which is the best choice? Here's what I think. In a perfect world, I'd want everyone to eat organic grass-fed meat and free-range poultry that's raised without growth hormones or antibiotics in environmentally friendly conditions. As for fish, I would love it if everyone could eat wild-caught rather than farmed fish. However, I know how expensive this kind of top-quality fare can be, especially if you have a family. It's actually hard for me in good conscience to recommend such an expensive choice (I'm the nutrition coach for all Americans, not just the rich ones!). I know that many of you reading this are watching every dollar while trying to get nutritious meals on the table three times a day for your families. You should have affordable options.

But I also feel strongly that high-quality meat, poultry, and fish are healthier than many of their affordable conventional counterparts. It's really astonishing to see the unpleasantness involved in the raising of conventional meat and farmed fish. And in my opinion, they have less of the good stuff that meat is supposed to contain and more of the bad stuff that it shouldn't.

Farmed fish are particularly disgusting. I don't want to gross you out, but they are often raised beneath suspended cages of chickens, where the fish feed on the feathers and feces that fall through the cages and into the water below (and in fish farms in China, it's pig feces). The vast majority of frozen fish in US supermarkets is raised this way in Asian countries, where standards and regulations are lower than in the United States. (To learn much more about how your food is produced and manufactured, I recommend reading *The Omnivore's Dilemma,* by Michael Pollan, or check out his Web site michaelpollan.com.)

On the question of how to best feed yourself and your family on a limited budget, here's what I recommend: Choose grass-fed meat when possible. A bit less costly than organic grass-fed meat, the antibiotic-free and grass-fed options are leaner and contain more nutrients than their conventional counterparts. Keep a watchful eye on sales and specials at your local grocery store and markets. Buy extra grass-fed meat on sale and freeze it for meals later in the week. As for poultry, when affordable, choose free-range birds, raised without antibiotics. Like grass-fed meat, antibiotic-free poultry is more nutritious and a healthier option than conventionally raised chicken.

Balance what you spend on meat and poultry by planning some less-expensive meatless meals that feature beans or eggs each week. You can also make meat an accompaniment to a meal rather than the main attraction. Think stir-fries, casseroles, soups, stews, tacos, even pizzas and omelets.

When protecting yourself and your family from the chemical assaults in the food supply, it's also a really good idea to avoid obesogens. These are chemicals in foods that make you fat by interrupting hormonal balance, which causes weight gain. They alter the regulatory system that controls your weight. Obesogens are found in meat, poultry, and fish treated with hormones and antibiotics and in produce fertilized with proteins and chemicals that disturb hormonal balance. To offset the effects of obesogens, eat organic peaches, plums, berries, oranges, apples, and bell peppers. When possible, eat free-range poultry, organic grass-fed meat, and wild-caught fish. Also buy and store food and beverages in BPA-free plastic containers. BPA (bisphenol A), an environmental obesogen found in plastic containers, has been linked to obesity by disrupting hormonal balance in the body and increasing fat cell size.

Enjoy eggs without worries of the past. For many years, nutrition experts thought that the cholesterol in eggs was bad for heart health; it was believed that dietary cholesterol raised cholesterol levels in the blood. Although it's true that high levels of LDL ("bad") cholesterol do boost cardiovascular disease risk, more recent research has taught us that cholesterol in foods such as egg yolks has only a weak impact on blood cholesterol levels. In fact, eggs contain a wide range of nutrients that are actually good for heart health. Egg yolks are loaded with minerals, including calcium and magnesium (both lacking in women), not to mention folate, vitamin B_6, and vitamins A and E. What's more, egg yolks provide carotenoids essential for healthy eyes, protecting against age-related macular degeneration. Studies show that for most people, eating a modest number of whole eggs/egg yolks has no negative effect on heart disease risk. That's why the F-15 Plan allows six whole eggs per week. (If you have heart disease or diabetes, check with your doctor, who may recommend sticking to three yolks a week.) As for egg whites, go ahead and have them when you want; they are an excellent source of protein. An egg's cholesterol is found in its yolk.

Hard-cooked eggs are an excellent high-protein addition to meals and snacks. You can save time by boiling them up by the dozen. Keep them in the fridge, and grab them when you need to add protein to a meal. Slice them into salads, chop them up and sprinkle them over cooked vegetables, or eat them as is with a sprinkle of paprika, chili powder, cumin, or whatever spices you enjoy. After you boil up a dozen, peel them all, slip them into a bag, and you're good to go. Peeled boiled eggs stay fresh in the refrigerator for up to 7 days. Here's how to hard-cook eggs: Place them in a single layer in a saucepan. Add water to cover the eggs by 1 inch. Turn the heat to high until they're just boiling. Remove them from the burner, cover them, and let them stand for 9 minutes (medium eggs), 12 minutes (large eggs), or 15 minutes (extra-large eggs). Rinse with cold water to cool them. Remember: The F-15 Plan limits egg yolks to six per week.

Studies show that for most people, eating a modest number of whole eggs/egg yolks has no negative affect on heart disease risk.

Go meatless sometimes. I'm okay with people who choose to eat a vegetarian or vegan diet. I choose to eat meat, poultry, and fish because I prefer them for taste, convenience, and especially for their delivery of important nutrients to the diet. However, I recognize the value of a diet that minimizes meat and focuses more on plants: vegetables, fruits, legumes, seeds, and grains. Even though I'm a carnivore, I believe we can all benefit from eating a little less meat and a great deal more plants. The mounting evidence of the health benefits associated with a plant-based diet that includes copious amounts of colorful vegetables and fruits and that uses whole, unprocessed grains is astounding. That's why I recommend going meatless for at least one meal once or twice a week, working your way up to several meatless meals per week. We surely want to enjoy the health benefits of eating more fruits and vegetables, including weight loss, youthful dewy skin, and longevity.

Don't forget about nuts! Nuts are a big part of the F-15 Plan. Not only are they rich in protein, but they also contain healthy fats that help to protect you from heart disease and other chronic illnesses. They're also good sources of nutrients such as magnesium, potassium, and vitamin E. According to the Harvard School of Public Health, people who eat nuts several times per week have a 30 to 50 percent lower risk of heart problems (myocardial infarction, sudden cardiac death, and cardiovascular disease) than those who don't. Other studies have found that people who replace some of the meat in their diets with plant-based proteins, such as nuts, gain less weight over time than those who don't.

Sure, you have to make sure you don't eat too many nuts. Just keep your eyes on the correct serving sizes. And be sure to eat a variety of nuts so you can get all of their health benefits. For now, here are the numbers of nuts per 1-ounce serving.

Almonds: 22	Peanuts: 28
Brazil nuts: 6 to 8	Pecans: 20 halves
Cashews: 18	Pistachios: 47 (shelled)
Hazelnuts (filberts): 20	Walnuts: 14 (halves)
Macadamia nuts: 10 to 12	

Q&A

TILAPIA AND FARMED FISH: WHAT YOU NEED TO KNOW

Q: **I've seen advertisements saying we should eat tilapia because it's the fish that was served at the Last Supper. Should I add tilapia to my grocery list?**

A: Absolutely not! Forget what the ads say. I don't think historians know definitively what was served at one of the holiest meals in history. But I'm pretty sure it wasn't anything like the tilapia available in most grocery stores and restaurants today. Some people speculate that because of the fish's aggressive breeding ability, it could have been a version of the fish we call tilapia that Jesus used to feed the five thousand as indicated in the Bible. However, tilapia is actually a class of several fish that originated in

Africa. It was brought to the United States because, again, it is a hearty fish that breeds and multiplies very quickly and is a bottom-feeder that basically can eat anything and survive. Today, this bottom-feeding scavenger fish is raised mostly in sea-cage fish farms and force-fed a diet that includes antibiotics, hormones, harmful chemicals, and animal feces. Plus, it's high in omega-6 fatty acids, which are not good for your brain or heart. Instead of this allegedly "holy" fish, choose wild Alaskan salmon, Alaska pollock, Atlantic cod, striped bass, haddock, rainbow trout, herring, flounder, sardines, blue crab, red and yellow snapper, Arctic char, sablefish, and albacore tuna.

FATS AND OILS

Fat and Oil Serving Sizes

FOOD	SERVING SIZE
Vegetable oil (canola, corn, olive, peanut, safflower, soybean, sunflower), butter, margarine, and mayonnaise	Oils, butter, trans fat–free buttery spread: 1 tablespoon—about the size of a poker chip
Salad dressing	2 tablespoons—looks like ¾ of a shot glass
Olives	4 large
Avocado	¼ fruit—about the size of two thumbs
Guacamole	¼ cup
Nuts (peanuts, almonds, pistachios, walnuts, pecans, etc.); note that nuts are also listed under Proteins	1 ounce—about the size of ½ a shot glass
Nut butters (peanut, pecan, almond, etc.); note that nut butters are also listed under Proteins	2 tablespoons—about the diameter of a Ping-Pong ball

Tips for Choosing Fats and Oils

Over the past two decades, we've been brainwashed into thinking that all fats are bad. But the truth is, some fats are actually quite good for us and are an important part of a healthy diet. Monounsaturated fats—the fats found in avocados, nuts, olives, and their oils—and polyunsaturated fats—the fats found in nuts, seeds, and some kinds of fish—are essential to good health, and they are linked to better health in your body and mind. Since fats help you to feel satiated, healthy fats are an important part of a smart weight-loss plan.

Choose cold-pressed oils. These oils are made without the use of heat or chemicals, which can destroy nutrients.

Throw away spoiled fats and oils. If an oil or high-fat food has an "off" smell, it may be rancid.

Select nuts and nut butters without added salt and sugar. Nuts are great for you, but the salty or sugary seasonings aren't. Store nuts and seeds in the freezer to prolong their shelf life and to protect them from becoming rancid.

Get friendly with avocados. You may not have grown up with this delicious fruit, but it is considered by many to be one of the world's healthiest foods. It contains healthy amounts of several nutrients, including folate, vitamin B_5, vitamin B_6, vitamin C, vitamin E, vitamin K, potassium, fiber, and small amounts of several other vitamins and minerals. It's also an excellent source of monounsaturated fats, which are associated with reduced risk of heart disease, eye disease, arthritis, and some kinds of cancer. Slice it into salads, mix it into smoothies, and mash it up as a delicious veggie dip or as a replacement for mayonnaise on sandwiches and in salads.

Go for guacamole. Buy it premade, or make your own by combining mashed avocado, chopped tomatoes, chopped red onion, lime juice or lemon juice, and a touch of garlic. Use it as a delicious dip for vegetables.

Tips for Choosing Grains and Breads

Whole grains are a good source of fiber, folate, B vitamins, and minerals such as iron, selenium, and magnesium. Eating high-fiber foods helps with weight loss because they fill you up, stave off hunger, and thus prevent you from overeating and filling up on undesirable high-fat, high-sodium, or sugar-laden foods. However, eating refined grains made of processed refined flour and sugar has the reverse effect on the body. Rather than providing the body with energy, the intended purpose for carbohydrates, refined grains are used up quickly by the body and converted to sugar in the blood, which not only causes weight gain but also defeats the purpose of eating them at all. Refined grains in the form of bread, cakes, cookies, crackers, biscuits, waffles, and pancakes can derail your weight-loss goals. Furthermore, even some wheat products can be a bane to the diets of people who are insulin-resistant. The secret to long-term weight loss is to eat whole grains strategically. This means that during the weight-loss process, it is important to limit the number of servings of these foods, exercise portion control, and choose them in their most natural, whole, and unprocessed state. Here are a few tips I'd like you to keep in mind.

Eat whole, sprouted grain breads and cereals. My absolute favorite bread is Ezekiel 4:9 sprouted grain bread. I've recommended it to so many people that I should be on the company's payroll! I consider Ezekiel to be one of the healthiest breads on the market today. Based on the Bible quote from, you guessed it, Ezekiel 4:9: "Take also unto thee wheat, and barley, and beans, and lentils and millet, and spelt and put them in one vessel," Ezekiel bread uses sprouted, whole, unprocessed grains and seeds. Sprouting allows these healthy ingredients to release their nutrients more slowly and easily. The Ezekiel brand uses no flour or refined sugar, just supernutritious, unprocessed sprouted grains. This

GRAINS AND BREADS
Grain and Bread Serving Sizes

FOOD	SERVING SIZE
Breads (bread, bagels, biscuits, corn-bread, English muffins, tortillas, etc.)	1 slice of bread—the size of a cassette tape or small iPhone
	1 small bagel—the diameter of the top of a tuna can
	Other bread products: 1-ounce portion
Whole grains (amaranth, barley, buck-wheat, bulgur, millet, quinoa, rice, etc.)	½ cup cooked—the size of a light bulb
Pasta	½ cup cooked (1 ounce dry)—the size of a light bulb
Oatmeal	½ cup cooked (1 ounce dry)
Pancakes and waffles	Pancakes and waffles: 1-ounce portion of either—the size of a 4-inch CD
Popcorn	3 cups air-popped
Ready-to-eat breakfast cereal	1 cup flakes or 1¼ cups puffed

whole grain bread contains 18 amino acids, including all nine essential amino acids. Because it's sprouted, it is easier for your body to digest and to absorb its vitamins and minerals. It contains no genetically modified organisms (GMOs) or artificial ingredients of any kind and is only 80 calories per one-slice serving, compared to 100 to 130 calories per serving for its whole grain counterparts.

Choose whole grain pasta and sides. Again, when grains are refined or processed, they lose fiber and important nutrients. When you buy grains—such as rice, pasta, couscous, and similar side dishes—check the label to make sure they are whole and unprocessed. If you haven't tried them yet, experiment with red quinoa, whole grain couscous, wild rice, and brown, black, or red rice.

Give your oatmeal a lift. For more fiber, choose rolled oats or steel-cut oats rather than the instant variety.

Cook extra grains for freezing. Extra quinoa, barley, oats, and other cooked grains can be frozen and reheated easily for side dishes or to add to soups or stews.

Avoid "white" grains. This includes white rice, white bread, white flour, and products made with them. As I mentioned, refined grains, including the flour that you may use to cook other foods, tend to raise blood sugar levels and are quickly converted to sugar in the blood, rather than being slowly absorbed and preserved for sustained energy.

Change the way you think about noodles. When I say "noodle," you probably think of egg noodles or wheat pasta. Think again! Instead of these empty carbohydrates, try black-bean pasta, which has only 17 grams of carbs, 12 grams of filling fiber, and 25 whopping grams of protein. It is made with only two ingredients—black beans and water. Other healthy, low-carb, high-protein options are kelp, soba, or buckwheat noodles and shirataki noodles, a no-carb, calorie-free Japanese noodle made from the konjac yam, which once eaten swells to over 17 percent of its volume and fills you up like no other noodle to date. Try shirataki noodles in stir-fries, a great option to which you can add lots of flavorful ingredients, including sauces like hoisin, teriyaki, or peanut sauce. These noodles take on the flavor of the dish in which they are prepared.

Don't bother going gluten-free. Unless you have celiac disease or non-celiac gluten intolerance, you don't have to adopt a gluten-free (GF) diet.

Eating GF is all the rage lately, but there isn't really any evidence that it helps you unless you have some kind of gluten disorder. What I like about the GF diet is that it directs you away from eating lots of wheat, but the downside is that many GF breads and grain products are low in fiber and full of sugar, excess fat, and refined rice flour. And they're expensive, too. Just about everyone should be eating fewer grains and more produce, but unless you have an intolerance for gluten, there's no reason to switch to a GF diet. Even those diagnosed with celiac disease or a gluten intolerance certainly do not have to buy GF-labeled products in a bag or box. Most are a waste of your hard-earned money. If you have to avoid gluten, stick to the whole foods that are naturally gluten-free.

In the Next Chapter: Phase 1 of the **F-15** Plan

We've done some very important work in this chapter. We've examined the 10 Success Strategies of the F-15 Plan. And we've gone over the optimal portion sizes for vegetables, fruits, proteins, dairy, fats, and grains. Now it's time to really dig in to the F-15 Plan. In the next chapter, we'll take a close look at Phase 1, which is structured to jump-start your metabolism and activate high-level fat-burning the minute you get started. I'll tell you about all of the delicious options for food that you'll have during Phase 1 and the reasons the choices you make will build a foundation for a lifetime of weight loss and better health. Plus, I'll give you meal plans, recipes, tracking tools, and loads of time-saving, money-saving tips that will help you to meet your goals.

Part II

THE **F-15** PLAN

Chapter 4

PHASE 1:
HIGH-INTENSITY FAT BURNING

*Set your intention each day on being better than
you were the day before.*
—Dr. Ro

Now it's time to really dig in to the F-15 Plan. You're ready to roll:
You're up to speed on serving sizes, and you understand all of the
thinking behind the F-15 Plan. Now it's time to start eating!

The F-15 Plan begins with a high-intensity fat-burning phase. During
this first phase of my three-phase plan, you'll eat in a way that primes
you for success. The serving strategy I've designed for Phase 1 optimizes
your body for high-intensity fat burning, weight loss, and detoxification
by helping you to replace empty-calorie junk food with the nutrients and
muscle-building power of whole foods. This is the phase that primes
your body for the weight loss that you came here for. During these first
15 days, you'll lay the foundation for continued success in this phase and
the phases that follow.

Phase 1 lasts for 15 days. After you complete Phase 1, you will then
progress to Phase 2, followed by Phase 3, with each phase lasting for
15 days. In the weeks and months that follow, if you want to lose more,
or if you want to build on the momentum you experienced in the first
phase, you can always cycle back through Phase 1 for as long as you
need to and then gradually progress to Phases 2 and 3 after having lost
the intended weight.

For now, though, we're starting with a 15-pound weight-loss goal.
And remember, you will always have the option of staying in Phase 1

Success Story

Brittany Hardman

19 pounds lost

6 inches lost from the waist

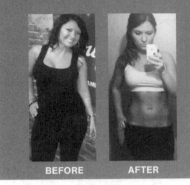

BEFORE   AFTER

Brittany was supermotivated to lose a few pounds. She was eager to lose 10 pounds—overnight, if possible. But who doesn't want that, right? Yeah, sure! Her problem was that she didn't know how to eat to live. Instead, she found herself eating for her taste buds and not for her life or for the body she said she wanted. This is a common misstep made by many of my clients; they say one thing but do another. They don't realize that what they say with their mouths must be consistent with what they think or tell themselves in their minds, feel in their hearts, and know to be true in their guts. So we had to get Brittany to see her inconsistency and change her behavior to doing, not just saying and never following those words through with corresponding action.

We needed to stoke Brittany's metabolic fires. My strategy was to "lean out" her body. That meant the F-15 Phase 1 plan was the way to go. It helped her to cut her calories, it kept her full, and—because she ate only lean protein sources and leafy greens for 3 weeks—she got the results we were going for.

We also boosted Brittany's metabolism by adding in exercise. She worked out using my 15-minute workout routines twice a day. I recommended that Brittany drink plenty of water. In fact, water was the only beverage she drank. She had been accustomed to drinking sweet tea. That was the first to go.

Brittany has a sweet tooth and thought that because she had only a few pounds to lose, she could still inhale doughnuts, honey and cinnamon buns, and red velvet cake. However, since abs are made in the kitchen, we had to replace those with fruit desserts once she transitioned to Phase 2. We started with baked apples with a dusting of cinnamon and a handful of chopped walnuts. She also snacked occasionally on a 2-inch square of dark chocolate made of 65 to 80 percent cacao.

Because Brittany loved to snack and was working out so hard, we added watermelon with chili powder and DIY peanut butter protein bars, but she mostly consumed slices of turkey, baby carrots, cherry tomatoes, and hummus for snacks. She loved the Zucchini Pizza Wedges (page 111).

Losing weight helped Brittany gain her confidence back. "I'm a single mom who has to set an example for my daughter. I had lost a little of myself until I saw my abs again. Before, I dreaded looking at myself in the mirror. Now, in my new body, looking in the mirror makes me happy!"

longer than 15 days if you choose to. This is your plan, and I've designed it to work for you in the ways that your body may need.

This first phase of the F-15 Plan will kick-start your weight loss and set your fat-burning factory on fire! Here's what you'll get in this chapter as you kick off Phase 1 of the F-15 Plan.

A 15-day serving plan: I'll give you specific guidelines that show you exactly how to allocate your 15 daily servings during this first 15-day phase.

A 15-day meal plan: The Phase 1 F-15 Meal Plan demonstrates ways that you can incorporate your daily servings into daily menus for 15 days. You don't have to follow my suggested meal plan; the F-15 Plan is all about you, so you can structure your meals however you like. But I find that many of my clients appreciate having a step-by-step plan to follow, so I am happy to provide one for you.

Supereasy, yummy recipes: For your convenience, I've created recipes for delicious, filling F-15 foods that fit perfectly into this phase. Many of them take only 15 minutes (or less) to prepare. I've kept your busy schedule top of mind.

15-minute moves: To move you toward your weight and health goals, I've designed some simple, effective 15-minute workouts that rev up your metabolism, build muscle, and help to burn fat fast.

Now, let's get you those servings!

The Phase 1 Servings Plan

The primary goal of this first phase of the F-15 Plan is to burn fat. We do this by including plenty of power-packed foods in each meal, including lean protein, nutrient-rich vegetables, low-fat dairy, and heart-protecting fats. Each day you'll eat 15 servings of foods that will help to kick-start weight loss and start moving your body into a leaner, cleaner state.

The food combinations in Phase 1 are designed to detoxify your body. By eliminating sugar, grains, fruit, alcohol, and fried or processed foods during this phase, you prime your body for weight loss and you gain the health benefits of optimum nutrition.

Think of yourself as returning to an almost embryonic state in which your body is becoming ready to receive all of the goodness that healthy food can provide. You will add some of those foods back in during later stages of the F-15 Plan, but for now, your body will benefit most from a detoxifying, super fat-burning approach to eating. Controlling portions and choosing high-impact foods will prime your digestive system to work its hardest, metabolizing and absorbing nutrients and feeding your body the fuel it needs to go the distance for you.

As you follow Phase 1 of the F-15 Plan, the foods you eat will help build muscle and rev up your metabolism. By adding in exercise, you'll stimulate your body to use the food you eat for energy rather than storing it as fat.

It's this simple: Each day during Phase 1 you'll eat a total of 15 servings of food: four servings of protein (lean meat, poultry, fish, beans, nuts, seeds, and eggs), six servings of nonstarchy "everyday" vegetables, two servings of low-fat dairy foods, and three servings of fat. That comes to a total of 15 servings per day.

BEHIND THE SERVINGS

I've carefully thought out the serving strategy of each phase of the F-15 Plan to make it as effective as possible yet simple and easy to follow. Still, I think it's helpful for you to have an idea of where my suggestions come from. So here's a quick explanation.

Protein: Eating adequate amounts of protein helps with weight loss in several ways. Studies show that protein helps the body keep appetite under control, and it contributes to an active and strong metabolism. Scientists have also found that people on higher-protein diets lose more

PHASE I SERVINGS

During Phase 1 of the F-15 Plan, you'll eat the following foods.

✓ **4** servings of protein

✓ **6** servings of Everyday Vegetables

✓ **2** servings of low-fat dairy

✓ **3** servings of fat

TOTAL: 15 servings per day

(For a full review of serving sizes, see the tables in Chapter 3.)

weight and more fat and preserve more muscle than those who follow lower-protein diets. For those reasons, you'll be eating four servings of protein daily in Phase 1 of the F-15 Plan. It's not just important to eat a certain amount of protein each day. Studies show that spreading your protein out *throughout* the day makes a difference. For example, a 2015 study published in the *American Journal of Clinical Nutrition* found that people who eat protein at each meal of the day lose more weight than those who don't. That's the reason you'll find protein included in most of your meals and snacks. Protein is the fuel that helps to keep your fat-burning metabolism machine going strong!

Vegetables: Just as protein helps you to feel satiated, so too do vegetables. Because they are high in fiber, veggies help fill you up and chase away hunger. Eat them at every meal and snack and you're unlikely to be hungry. Keep in mind that there are two kinds of vegetables on the F-15 Plan: Everyday Vegetables and Occasional Vegetables. Everyday Vegetables are exactly what they sound like—vegetables that you can eat throughout the day, every day. These vegetables are high in fiber and nutrients and low in calories and carbohydrates. In Phase 1, you can eat six servings a day of Everyday Vegetables; in later phases, you'll eat four or five servings daily. Occasional Vegetables are higher in calories and carbohydrates, so they're limited to two servings a week in Phase 2 and Phase 3. I leave them out of Phase 1 because, remember, we're trying to optimize your body for fat burn, metabolic power, and weight loss during this phase. For a full list of Everyday Vegetables and Occasional Vegetables, see pages 56 to 57 in Chapter 3.

In addition to being an important part of your dining experience during Phase 1 of the F-15 Plan, Everyday Vegetables are your go-to food when you get hungry between meals. I recommend six servings of Everyday Vegetables per day in Phase 1, but it is okay to add an additional serving or two each day if you need a little extra food.

Low-fat dairy: When you drink your milk or eat yogurt or cheese, you're getting calcium, which has been shown to help with weight loss. In fact, some studies have found that people who include calcium-rich, low-fat dairy foods in their weight-loss programs are more likely to succeed than those who don't. Calcium appears to help increase fat burn and boosts metabolism. And low-fat dairy foods include two satiating ingredients: protein plus a bit of fat, which help you feel fuller longer. For those reasons, I include two daily servings of dairy in each phase of the F-15 Plan.

Fat: It sounds hard to believe since we were told that "fat makes us fat" for so many years, but in reasonable amounts, fat actually helps to make us thin because it is satiating, filling, and helps to prevent hunger. That said, fat is the diet's most concentrated source of energy and is needed for the absorption of fat-soluble vitamins A, D, E, and K. Essentially we need fat to burn fat. Obviously, too much fat *will* contribute to making you fat. But three servings a day, as I recommend in each phase of the F-15 Plan, can go a long way toward helping you cut back on excess food without feeling hungry, not to mention the important contribution to health benefits, including your weight loss.

SUPER TIME-SAVERS

If you're not used to doing very much cooking, you may be concerned about the effort involved in creating healthy meals and snacks. I get it: It's absolutely easier to hit the drive-thru than to prepare a meal at home. But hitting the drive-thru hasn't been working so well for you, has it? Remember, you want to change your body, and that means changing your everyday cooking habits. The good news is that by taking a few simple steps, you can save time (and money). Here are some food prep tips that will get you in and out of the kitchen fast.

Combine your prep work. To save time throughout the week, schedule a weekly veggie-prep night. Put on some amazing music and spend 15 minutes washing, cutting, and storing the week's produce in airtight clear glass or BPA-free plastic containers. To save time in the morning, make big batches of oatmeal, divide into servings, pour into resealable plastic bags, and freeze for a grab-and-go breakfast. When you're ready to eat, remove the oatmeal from the bag, place it in a microwaveable bowl, and heat until ready.

Cook extra for leftovers. When making dinner (during the week), make three or four extra servings and freeze them to have on other days. And save time on veggie sides and mains. Steam, sauté, and stir-fry veggies in batches ahead of time, and freeze or refrigerate them for weekly meals and sides. Roast a big pan of veggies, and save the leftovers in airtight clear glass or plastic containers in the fridge.

Stay organized. Shop once a week for perishable items and once a month for staples; buy in bulk to save money. Keep your fridge, cabinets, and pantry organized

WATCH THESE PHASE I DIET TRAPS

Certain foods are not included in this phase of the F-15 Plan. That's because they interfere with the goals in this phase: high-intensity fat burn, optimal metabolism revving, detoxification, and losing weight without triggering cravings and hunger. Here's why I suggest skipping the following foods during the next 15 days.

Added sugar: Sugar is added to almost everything. You know it's in soda, candy, desserts, sugary breakfast cereals, waffles, pancakes, and other sweet foods. But it's also in some unlikely places, including certain prepared salad dressings, pasta sauces, soups, breads, frozen meals,

for easy access to ingredients you use regularly. To increase produce intake, store it at eye-level in the refrigerator. Toss one Bluapple into each of your produce bins to extend the shelf life of your produce. These small apple-shaped produce savers absorb the ethylene gas that producers use to speed up the ripening process. Replacing the removable tab on a monthly basis will not only keep your produce fresh but also help you to save your hard-earned money on food you will no longer have to throw out because it matured too quickly.

Stock up. Whenever possible, buy in bulk for staples such as canned tuna, salmon, canned or dried beans, peas, dried nuts, and seeds once a month. For meat, chicken, and fish, separate large quantities into individual servings and freeze for easy use.

Shop the sales. Take advantage of sales on fresh fruits and vegetables. Wash, cut, and then pack produce in freezer bags in individual or family-size servings to pop into a sauté pan with a little extra virgin olive oil and a cup of water for weeknight dinners (for leafy greens, blanch for a few minutes in water before freezing them). You can also freeze produce to save time on smoothies. Always keep produce cut and stored in bags in the freezer or in airtight glass or plastic bowls in the fridge for smoothies and juices.

This may seem overwhelming at first. But once you start seeing results on the scale and on your waistline, you'll be excited to get your food prep done every week.

canned and frozen fruit, barbecue sauce, even some kinds of pizza! Sure, sugar tastes good. But it works against you when you want to lose weight, not only because it contains loads of empty calories but also because the more sugar you eat, the more you want.

When you eat foods that contain sugar, your body reacts by releasing the extra insulin needed to move sugar from your blood to your cells. Right after eating sugar, your blood sugar goes way up; not long after a blood sugar spike, your blood sugar falls rapidly. When this sudden fall occurs, your body responds by causing you to crave even more sugar! It's an endless cycle that just keeps taking you from one sweets craving to the next. Over time, your pancreas can have trouble making enough insulin, and in the process, you increase your risk of developing diabetes.

If you can stop eating sugar for a while, something wonderful happens: You actually start craving less sugar. So just as eating more sugar makes you *want* more sugar, eating less sugar makes you *want* less sugar. That's why I don't include any added sugar in this phase of the F-15 Plan. I don't even include fruit in Phase 1 because the natural sugar in fruit can interfere with your initial ability to shake off added-sugar habits and cravings. Later, when you're in better control of your sugar intake and your cravings have subsided, you can have fruit and even an occasional sweet treat. But for this 15-day phase, I urge you to cut out all sugar. Before you know it—in as little as a couple of days—you'll find it easier and easier to forego sugar. Won't it be a relief not to be tied to constant sugar cravings?

Fruit: Fruit is an important part of your diet because it provides lots of essential nutrients, such as vitamins, minerals, antioxidants, and phytochemicals, not to mention both soluble and insoluble fiber. Fruit also contains varying amounts of natural sugar. Some fruits have more than others: Berries are lower in sugar, and bananas are higher in sugar, for example. By no means is the sugar found in fruit the same as the sugar found in, say, a piece of chocolate cake or a cookie. Fructose, or fruit sugar, actually contributes to sustained energy. One study found that bananas triggered a greater shift in dopamine during intense cycling compared to a sports drink. So don't get me wrong here, including fruit in your diet adds to your well-being; it doesn't detract from it. The reason I've removed it from the first phase of your meal plan is that I want you to start from ground zero. In Phases 2 and 3, you will get to enjoy the sweet benefits of eating fruit. That's a promise.

Grains: I recommend skipping grains during Phase 1 because you are more likely to lose weight quickly without grains, which are higher in calories than vegetables. While whole grains do contain healthy nutrients and fiber, many are also converted to sugars, which can remind your body of what you want it to forget right now—its reliance on sugar. Grains come back into the plan in Phase 3.

Alcohol: There are a few reasons I recommend skipping wine, beer, and other alcohol during Phase 1 of the F-15 Plan. Let's start with detoxing. This phase is focused on removing the effects of empty-calorie foods on your body, which will allow your gastrointestinal system to start fresh, so to speak. Alcohol, like sugar, can be toxic to the body. Excessive alcohol drinking—more than one drink per day (for women) and more than two drinks per day (for men)—increases the risk of cancers of the mouth, tongue, esophagus, and stomach. Researchers believe that the reasons may be associated with the distillation process of the alcohol in all its forms. Also, alcohol can have a bloating effect on the body, the exact opposite of what you wish to do to your body as you work to achieve your desired results.

Secondly, alcohol is not included in this phase because it is 7 empty calories per gram, which is like having a little pat of butter in a shot glass. Alcoholic beverages provide no nutritional support. To ensure that you get the biggest weight-loss results, your calories are reserved for the foods that offer the greatest nutritional content and health benefits, without the extra calories

As you journey to losing the weight for the last time, it is important to focus on consistently putting the right foods in your body to support your goals, not sabotage them.

Now that I've shared my two primary reasons for skipping alcohol during your Phase 1 experience, here's the third. Drinking alcohol can weaken your resolve to stay on a healthy meal program like the F-15 Plan. Drinking can cause you to relax your defenses, which often makes dieters more likely to adopt a kind of "might as well" philosophy. Well, since I cheated on that, I "might as well" drink this. You see where I'm going here? In my business, I've seen a drink here or there on a diet lead to eating more salty snacks, sweets, and other foods. You know, the ones you're trying to wean yourself off of during this phase. But don't take my word for it. There's this: In one British study, researchers found that when 80 dieters kept food diaries and recorded the foods that lured them into lapses for 1 week, alcohol was their biggest temptation. It was the calorie source most responsible for taking them off course, away from the diet they *said* they would stick to in order to lose weight. It turns out that dieters give in more frequently—as much as half the time—to alcohol than all manner of sugary and salty and fatty snacks. They also tend to underestimate liquid calories, and their bodies pay less attention to them. So it's easy to consume a few hundred calories during cocktail hour and have just as big an appetite at dinner as you would have had without the drinks.

Finally, there's one more reason. Alcohol contains sugar, and some drinks—especially cocktails made with fruit juice, soda, and sugary syrup—are chock-full of sugar and the empty calories that sugar contains. Believe it or not, a 12-ounce can of cola contains about 10 teaspoons of sugar.

Since breaking your sugar addiction (or preference, again, I don't judge) is a goal in Phase 1, it's best to avoid alcohol as you set yourself free from the circular hold that sugar may have on you. Listen, this makes sense. We are social beings at our core, and we enjoy socializing with a glass of wine, a bottle of bear, or a colorful cocktail. I'm not saying you can't ever drink again—you can, in later phases of the F-15 Plan. But for now, I hope you'll commit to leaving alcohol on the shelf for at least 15 to 30 days. You might choose to leave it on the shelf for a lot longer once you see the results of your hard work on this plan!

However, if you *must* have a drink despite the sound reasons that I've laid out for you, I propose that you wait until you achieve your desired results during the first two phases and have your drink in Phase 3. Should you decide to drink, choose low-calorie options, such as wine, champagne (a 6-ounce serving is only 90 calories), light beer, or hard liquor mixed with seltzer water. Limit yourself to no more than two drinks per week, and avoid sugary mixed drinks. (A margarita can have as much as 540 calories, but a 1-ounce shot of tequila has only about 70.) For every alcoholic drink you consume, have one or two glasses of water to prevent dehydration. And start the next day with my Pick-Me-Up Green Smoothie recipe in Phase 2 (page 171) to help restore any lost nutrients.

Processed foods: If I had my way, you would avoid highly processed foods altogether. They are stuffed with excess fat (especially low-quality, saturated or, worse yet, trans fats), added sugar, salt, artificial colors and additives, and other additives our bodies would be a lot better off without. I understand that in a time-starved world with so many demands on your schedule, it seems that processed foods are the easiest choice. I offer you this: If you plan ahead—as you'll learn to do in this book—you

SUPPLEMENTS TO TAKE EVERY DAY

As you begin following the F-15 Plan, I recommend that you take a daily multivitamin and a daily probiotic supplement. Here's why.

Daily multivitamin: Even though you'll be eating a highly nutritious diet on the F-15 Plan, your body may need a little extra boost of vitamins and minerals. That's why it's a good idea to take a daily multivitamin. It's like an insurance policy; you just want to make sure that you're getting enough of the essential nutrients in the proper quantities your body requires for its normal functions, particularly for all that you're asking of it right now. I recommend the SuperNutrition brand. Choose the SimplyOne Women if you're a woman under 50 or SimplyOne 50+ Women for women 50 and over. These options are also available to men with SuperNutrition's men's blends. These vitamins are available at health food stores or online.

Probiotics: We think of bacteria as being harmful to our bodies. But our guts are actually teeming with a mix of "good" and helpful "bad" bacteria that facilitate digestion of the foods we eat and absorption of their nutrients. Probiotic supplements are made of natural good bacteria that balance the mix of those bacteria naturally found in the gut and that with aging, change of diet, and some medications become unbalanced. Yogurt with live, active cultures and kefir (a tart, yogurt-like drink made of cow's or goat's milk) are two examples of natural probiotic-containing foods. I recommend taking a daily probiotic supplement because probiotics boost your digestive health, balance "good" and "bad" bacteria in your gut, help your body to improve carbohydrate metabolism and absorb nutrients better, and move stool through your intestinal tract more effectively. Probiotics are not laxatives, but when you first start taking them, you'll probably notice that your stool is bulkier and more voluminous. This is good, because it's proof that your body is detoxifying and naturally revving up your digestive system to work more effectively for you. My fave probiotic supplement is Align. I recommend it to my clients as a matter of course.

Success Story

Susan Moore

20.2 pounds lost
6.3 inches lost overall

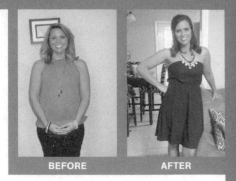

BEFORE   AFTER

Susan is a busy professional who found that working 14-hour days, putting family and career first, and having no time left for herself or to go to the gym meant gaining a few extra pounds. In her forties, she noticed her metabolism slowing down, and losing weight became more difficult. Susan came to me to reboot her life and to help her shed about 15 excess pounds.

When I first met Susan, she didn't drink water; she drank sweet tea. In Alabama, sweet tea is like water. It's *the* go-to drink for Alabamians, who drink it by the quart. The food culture and foodscape here is not exactly heart-healthy, and Susan, though a mostly lean person for much of her life, was unaware that her eating habits were not healthy. Because she had not had to worry about it before, she didn't realize the effect that her environment had on her food choices.

To change Susan's eating habits, we started with incorporating more vegetables and fruits into her diet, which is the hallmark of the F-15 Plan. Eating this way not only gave her weight loss a boost but also helped speed up her metabolism. In Susan's case, we switched her brown-and-beige, meat-and-potatoes (with gravy) diet to a more colorful, healthier fruit- and veggie-rich diet with fewer calories, more fiber (to keep her fuller for longer periods of time during her long work hours), and greater health benefits.

Susan dines out a lot because of her job. In Susan's area of Alabama, there are lots of chain restaurants happy to serve huge, oversize portions, so she began to ask up front for take-home bags. She had the server split entrées in half, pack one half in a to-go bag, and serve the other on her plate. This was a big step for her because the servers with their Southern hospitality didn't "take too kindly" to this treatment at first. After all, the South is not a place where people turn down food.

Instead of alcohol or sweet tea, Susan chose water with fresh cucumber, lemon, or lime, but on special occasions, she had one white wine spritzer to sip (easy on the wine, heavy on the soda water). Susan's changes in eating habits, combined with taking small walks in the morning and fitting in 15-minute workouts after work about three times per week, helped her to lose 20 pounds and over 6 inches from her small frame.

"I learned to live without making food the center of my life on this plan," Susan says. "Now when I eat out, I choose lean protein and a salad, not the two meats and three sides that I used to get."

won't need to rely on heavily processed foods that you'd rather not feed to yourself and your family in the first place.

The Phase 1 **F-15** Meal Plan

As I've discussed, this first phase of the F-15 Plan includes four servings of protein, six servings of vegetables, two servings of low-fat dairy, and three servings of fat. Although I recommend having protein and vegetables at each meal and snack, the way you choose to allocate your daily servings is purely up to you. Some people find it more convenient to design their own daily plans—if that's you, all the better! Just know that I've done the heavy lifting for you so that you don't have to rack your brain to figure out what's for dinner, or any meal for that matter. The F-15 Plan is designed with your needs and weight-loss goals in mind. I've created 15 days of tasty meal plans to help you succeed at losing the weight, now that you've gotten on board and lost the "wait." You can follow them every day, once in a while, or not at all; it's totally up to you. As long as you stick with the Phase 1 servings plan, you're good to go!

PHASE I, WEEK I

Notes about the Meal Plans

- Meal plans include approximately 1,200 to 1,400 calories per day.
- Foods listed in **bold** have recipes in the recipe section.
- Asterisks (*) denote there is a variation in the ingredient and/or its amount for that recipe for that specific meal and day.
- Have lemon water with each meal and snack. Lemon water is made with water and the juice of two lemon wedges. Mint lemon water is made by adding 2 tablespoons chopped fresh mint. Basil lemon water is made by adding 2 tablespoons chopped fresh basil. Cucumber lemon water is made by adding 3 to 5 slices cucumber. Or you can mix any combination of these herbs with lemon and/or cucumber for a refreshing drink.

Day I

MEAL OR SNACK	FOODS	F-15 SERVINGS
Breakfast	1 serving **Prosciutto Breakfast Salad** (page 110) 1 cup green tea 16 ounces lemon water	1 Protein 2 Vegetables 1 Fat
Morning Snack	1 serving **Zucchini Pizza Wedges** (page 111) (use ¾ of sausage link) 20 ounces lemon water	¾ Protein 1 Vegetable 1 Dairy
Lunch	Spinach Salad with Broiled Salmon (4 ounces salmon, broiled, over salad made with 2 cups fresh spinach and ½ cup cherry tomatoes, tossed with 2 tablespoons fat-free Italian dressing) 20 ounces lemon water	1 Protein 2 Vegetables 1 Fat
Afternoon Snack	Turkey and Cheese Lettuce Wraps (1 ounce low-fat cheddar or Colby cheese, 1 ounce roast turkey breast, and 1 teaspoon mustard divided and wrapped in 2 leaves leaf lettuce) 20 ounces lemon water	¼ Protein 1 Dairy
Dinner	Black Bean Pasta with Chicken Breast and Sautéed Veggies (2 ounces boneless, skinless chicken breast, cut into strips, sautéed in 1 tablespoon extra virgin olive oil with ½ cup broccoli florets; 1 clove garlic, chopped; ¼ cup chopped tomatoes; and 1 tablespoon chopped fresh basil and served over 2 ounces black bean spaghetti, cooked according to package instructions, and topped with ½ tablespoon grated Parmesan cheese) 16 ounces lemon water	1 Protein 1 Vegetable 1 Fat
Evening Snack	20 ounces lemon water	
	Total for the Day	4 Proteins 6 Vegetables 2 Dairy 3 Fats

Day 2

MEAL OR SNACK	FOODS	F-15 SERVINGS
Breakfast	Veggie Egg Scramble (1 whole egg and 1 egg white scrambled with ½ cup chopped mushrooms, 1 tablespoon chopped onion, ½ cup chopped bell peppers, and 2 cups fresh spinach) 2 ounces extra-lean Canadian bacon, broiled with 1 spray olive oil cooking spray 1 cup 1% milk 1 cup green tea 16 ounces lemon water	1½ Proteins 2 Vegetables 1 Dairy ½ Fat
Morning Snack	Crudités with Pine Nut Hummus (½ cup baby carrots; 1 stalk celery, cut into thirds; ½ cup cherry tomatoes; and 2 tablespoons Sabra Roasted Pine Nut Hummus) 20 ounces lemon water	½ Protein 1 Vegetable
Lunch	1 serving **Lunchtime Turkey Rolls** (page 112) 1 cup green tea 20 ounces lemon water	1 Protein 1 Vegetable 1 Dairy 1 Fat
Afternoon Snack	20 ounces lemon water	
Dinner	1 serving **15-Minute Fish with Cucumber Sauce** (page 113) 12 spears asparagus, steamed Tossed Salad (2 cups mixed greens and ¼ cup cherry tomatoes, tossed with 1 tablespoon extra virgin olive oil and 2 tablespoons white balsamic vinegar) 20 ounces lemon water	1 Protein 2 Vegetables ½ Fat
Evening Snack	22 raw almonds 20 ounces lemon water	1 Fat
	Total for the Day	4 Proteins 6 Vegetables 2 Dairy 3 Fats

Day 3

MEAL OR SNACK	FOODS	F-15 SERVINGS
Breakfast	Cinnamon- and Mint-Topped Yogurt	2 Proteins
	(4 ounces low-fat plain yogurt topped with 1 tablespoon chopped fresh mint and ⅛ teaspoon ground cinnamon)	1 Dairy
	1 Aidells Organic Chicken and Apple Sausage, broiled	
	2 hard-cooked egg whites	
	½ cup 1% milk	
	1 cup green tea	
	16 ounces lemon water	
Morning Snack	Hummus-Stuffed Celery Sticks (Spread 1 tablespoon hummus on 2 stalks celery)	½ Vegetable
	20 ounces lemon water	
Lunch	Tossed Salad with Tuna	1 Protein
	(2 cups mixed greens, ¼ cup sliced mushrooms, ¼ cup grated carrots, and 1 cup halved cherry tomatoes tossed with 2 tablespoons fat-free Italian dressing and topped with 3 ounces drained canned water-packed tuna)	2½ Vegetables
	20 ounces lemon water	
Afternoon Snack	Cottage Cheese with Fresh Basil and Tomato	½ Vegetable
	(½ cup 1% cottage cheese mixed with ¼ tablespoon chopped fresh basil and 1 small plum tomato, sliced, drizzled with ¾ tablespoon extra virgin olive oil)	1 Dairy
		1 Fat
	20 ounces lemon water	
Dinner	*Chicken with Tomatoes and Olives, Steamed Cauliflower, and Sautéed Spinach	1 Protein
	(4 ounces boneless, skinless chicken breast, cut into strips, sautéed with ½ plum tomato, chopped; 2 tablespoons chopped onion; 1 tablespoon chopped olives; 2 tablespoons fat-free Italian dressing; ⅓ tablespoon dried basil; and 1 teaspoon dried oregano)	2½ Vegetables
		2 Fats
	Steamed cauliflower (⅓ cup cauliflower florets, steamed)	
	Sautéed spinach (2 cups fresh spinach sautéed in 1⅓ tablespoons extra virgin olive oil)	
	20 ounces lemon water	
Evening Snack	20 ounces lemon water	
	Total for the Day	4 Proteins
		6 Vegetables
		2 Dairy
		3 Fats

Day 4

MEAL OR SNACK	FOODS	F-15 SERVINGS
Breakfast	Peanut Butter Smoothie (1 cup 1% milk, 1 tablespoon peanut butter, ⅓ cup whey-based protein powder, and 3 ice cubes) 1 cup green tea 20 ounces lemon water	1 Protein 1 Dairy ½ Fat
Morning Snack	1 serving **Smoked Trout and Cottage Cheese Sliders** (page 114) 20 ounces lemon water	1 Protein 1 Vegetable 1 Dairy
Lunch	Spinach Salad with Tuna (2 cups fresh spinach, 1 ounce canned artichokes, ½ cup chopped tomato, 1 cooked egg white, chopped, and ½ cup sliced mushrooms tossed in 1 tablespoon balsamic vinegar and 1 tablespoon extra virgin olive oil and topped with 3 ounces drained canned water-packed tuna) 20 ounces lemon water	1 Protein 2 Vegetables 1 Fat
Afternoon Snack	Crudités with Pine Nut Hummus (½ cup baby carrots, ½ cup cherry tomatoes, and 1 tablespoon Sabra Roasted Pine Nut Hummus) 20 ounces lemon water	¼ Protein 1 Vegetable
Dinner	Stir-Fried Chicken and Vegetables over Spaghetti Squash (4 ounces boneless, skinless chicken breast, cut into strips; ½ cup broccoli florets; 3 tablespoons chopped onion; ¼ cup sliced mushrooms;1 teaspoon dried rosemary; and 1 teaspoon dried thyme stir-fried in 1 tablespoon extra virgin olive oil and served over ⅓ cup cooked spaghetti squash) 20 ounces lemon water	1 Protein 2 Vegetables 1½ Fats
Evening Snack	20 ounces lemon water	
	Total for the Day	4 Proteins 6 Vegetables 2 Dairy 3 Fats

Day 5

MEAL OR SNACK	FOODS	F-15 SERVINGS
Breakfast	Veggie Black Bean Breakfast Bowl	2 Proteins
	(4 tablespoons drained canned black beans; ½ cup chopped cauliflower florets; 1 cup fresh spinach; ½ cup chopped tomatoes; 1 clove garlic, chopped; 1 tablespoon chopped onion; 1 tablespoon chopped scallion; ½ tablespoon chopped fresh basil; and ½ tablespoon fresh thyme sautéed in ½ tablespoon extra virgin olive oil and then scrambled with 1 egg and 2 egg whites and topped with ¼ avocado, sliced)	1½ Vegetables 1 Fat
	1 cup green tea and 20 ounces lemon water	
Morning Snack	Warm Sun-Dried Tomato Pesto Breakfast Bowl	1 Dairy
	(Mix ¼ ounce warmed Classico Sun-Dried Tomato Pesto into 1 container [5.3 ounces] nonfat plain Greek yogurt)	
	20 ounces lemon water	
Lunch	Shrimp Power Veggie Salad	1 Protein
	(4.5 ounces cooked shrimp, ½ cup mixed greens, ½ cup fresh spinach, ½ cup broccoli florets, ½ cup halved cherry tomatoes, and 2 tablespoons fresh basil leaves tossed with 1 teaspoon mustard, 1 tablespoon extra virgin olive oil, and 2 tablespoons balsamic vinegar)	1 Vegetable 1 Fat
	20 ounces lemon water	
Afternoon Snack	Crudités and Cottage Cheese	½ Vegetable
	(½ cup 1% cottage cheese and ½ cup chopped carrots or celery)	1 Dairy
	20 ounces lemon water	
Dinner	Baked Fish with Sautéed Veggies	1 Protein
	Baked fish (dust 6 ounces haddock with garlic powder; top with a squeeze of lemon, 3 sprigs fresh dill, and 1 teaspoon trans–fat free buttery spread; wrap in parchment paper; and bake)	3 Vegetables 1 Fat
	Sautéed veggies (1 tablespoon chopped onion; ½ cup chopped zucchini; 1 Italian tomato, chopped; 1 teaspoon chopped fresh thyme; and 2 tablespoons chopped fresh basil sautéed in 2 teaspoons trans fat–free buttery spread)	
	Tossed Salad (2 cups mixed greens tossed with 2 tablespoons fat-free Italian dressing)	
	20 ounces lemon water	
Evening Snack	20 ounces lemon water	
	Total for the Day	4 Proteins 6 Vegetables 2 Dairy 3 Fats

Day 6

MEAL OR SNACK	FOODS	F-15 SERVINGS
Breakfast	1 serving **Tuscan Breakfast Salad with Canadian Bacon** (page 108) 1 cup 1% milk 1 cup green tea 16 ounces lemon water	2 Proteins 1½ Vegetables 1 Dairy 1 Fat
Morning Snack	Spiced Cottage Cheese Logs (2 stalks celery spread with ½ cup 1% cottage cheese mixed with ¼ teaspoon chili powder) 20 ounces lemon water	½ Vegetable 1 Diary
Lunch	Chicken Salad on a Bed of Mixed Greens (3 ounces cooked boneless, skinless chicken breast, cut into chunks, mixed with 1 stalk celery, diced; 3 tablespoons chopped onion; ¼ cup chopped bell pepper; 1 tablespoon coconut oil; and 1 tablespoon lemon juice, served over 1 cup mixed greens and ½ cup chopped baby kale and topped with ¼ teaspoon paprika and ¼ teaspoon ground black pepper) 20 ounces lemon water	1 Protein 2 Vegetables 1 Fat
Afternoon Snack	Turkey Lettuce Wraps (1 ounce roast turkey breast and 2 teaspoons mustard divided and wrapped in 2 leaves leaf lettuce) 20 ounces lemon water	¼ Protein
Dinner	Garlic-Rosemary Salmon with Sautéed Zucchini and Mushrooms Garlic-rosemary salmon (top 3 ounces salmon with 3 teaspoons minced garlic, ⅛ teaspoon each salt and ground black pepper, squeeze of lemon juice from 3 lemon wedges, 2 tablespoons fresh rosemary, and ½ tablespoon extra virgin olive oil and broil) Sautéed zucchini and mushrooms (½ cup sliced zucchini, ½ cup sliced mushrooms, and 1 tablespoon chopped onion sautéed in ½ tablespoon extra virgin olive oil) Tossed Salad (2 cups mixed greens tossed with 2 tablespoons fat-free Italian dressing) 20 ounces lemon water	1 Protein 2 Vegetables 1 Fat
Evening Snack	20 ounces lemon water	
	Total for the Day	4 Proteins 6 Vegetables 2 Dairy 3 Fats

Day 7

MEAL OR SNACK	FOODS	F-15 SERVINGS
Breakfast	Cinnamon- and Nut-Topped Yogurt	1 Protein
	(1 container [5.3 ounces] low-fat plain Greek yogurt mixed with ¼ teaspoon ground cinnamon and 1¼ tablespoons chopped walnuts)	1 Dairy 1 Fat
	1 hard-cooked egg	
	1 cup green tea	
	20 ounces lemon water	
Morning Snack	Guacamole and Crudités	1½ Vegetables
	Guacamole (¼ cup pureed avocado; 1 clove garlic, minced; and 1 ounce lemon juice)	1 Fat
	Crudités (2 carrots, cut into thirds; 1½ stalks celery, cut into thirds; and ⅛ cup sliced radishes)	
	20 ounces lemon water	
Lunch	Tuna Salad	1 Protein
	(3 ounces yellowfin tuna, grilled or baked, over 2 cups mixed greens tossed in ½ tablespoon extra virgin olive oil and the juice of 3 lemon wedges)	1 Vegetable ½ Fat
	20 ounces lemon water	
Afternoon Snack	Turkey Lettuce Wraps	1 Protein
	(3 ounces roast turkey breast and 2 teaspoons mustard divided and wrapped in 3 leaves butterhead lettuce)	½ Vegetable
	20 ounces lemon water	
Dinner	Broiled Halibut with Baked Vegetables	1 Protein
	(4 ounces halibut broiled with the juice of ½ lemon and 1 tablespoon extra virgin olive oil; melt ½ teaspoon trans fat–free buttery spread and mix with 1 tablespoon white balsamic vinegar and 2 tablespoons Worcestershire sauce; pour sauce over 12 spears asparagus and ½ cup broccoli florets and bake in a covered baking dish until bright green and tender)	3 Vegetables 1 Dairy ½ Fat
	Tossed Salad (1 cup mixed greens tossed with 2 tablespoons fat-free Italian dressing)	
	20 ounces lemon water	
Evening Snack	20 ounces lemon water	
	Total for the Day	4 Proteins 6 Vegetables 2 Dairy 3 Fats

PHASE I, WEEK 2

Day I

MEAL OR SNACK	FOODS	F-15 SERVINGS
Breakfast	Veggie Egg Scramble	2 Proteins
	(2 eggs scrambled in 1 tablespoon extra virgin olive oil with ½ cup sliced mushrooms, 1 tablespoon chopped onion, ½ cup chopped bell peppers, and 1 cup fresh spinach)	2 Vegetables
		1 Fat
	2 ounces extra-lean Canadian bacon, broiled with 1 spray olive oil cooking spray	
	1 cup green tea	
	16 ounces lemon water	
Morning Snack	Cottage Cheese and Crudités	1 Vegetable
	(½ cup 1% cottage cheese, ½ cup baby carrots, 3 stalks celery, and 5 cherry tomatoes, halved)	1 Dairy
	20 ounces lemon water	
Lunch	1 serving **Lunchtime Turkey Rolls** (page 112)	1 Protein
	1 cup green tea	1 Vegetable
	20 ounces lemon water	1 Dairy
Afternoon Snack	20 ounces mint lemon water	
Dinner	1 serving **15-Minute Fish with Cucumber Sauce** (page 113)	1 Protein
	12 spears asparagus, steamed	2 Vegetables
	Tossed Salad (1½ cups mixed greens; ½ cup cherry tomatoes; and ¼ avocado, sliced, tossed with 2 tablespoons fat-free Italian dressing)	1 Fat
	20 ounces lemon water	
Evening Snack	22 almonds	1 Fat
	20 ounces lemon water	
	Total for the Day	4 Proteins
		6 Vegetables
		2 Dairy
		3 Fats

Day 2

MEAL OR SNACK	FOODS	F-15 SERVINGS
Breakfast	Cinnamon- and Mint-Topped Yogurt	2 Proteins
	(4 ounces low-fat plain yogurt topped with 1 table-spoon chopped fresh mint and ⅛ teaspoon ground cinnamon)	1½ Dairy
	1 Aidells Organic Chicken and Apple Sausage, broiled	
	2 hard-cooked egg whites	
	1 cup 1% milk	
	1 cup green tea	
	16 ounces lemon water	
Morning Snack	20 ounces lemon water	
Lunch	Tossed Salad with Tuna	1 Protein
	(2 cups mixed greens, ½ cup sliced mushrooms, ½ cup grated carrots, and 1 cup halved cherry toma-toes tossed in 2 tablespoons fat-free Italian dressing and topped with 3 ounces drained canned water-packed tuna)	3 Vegetables
	20 ounces lemon water	
Afternoon Snack	Cottage Cheese with Fresh Basil and Tomato	½ Vegetable
	(¼ cup 1% cottage cheese mixed with ¼ tablespoon chopped fresh basil, and 1 small tomato, sliced, drizzled with ¾ tablespoon extra virgin olive oil)	½ Dairy
		¾ Fat
	20 ounces lemon water	
Dinner	*Stir-Fried Chicken with Tomatoes and Olives, Steamed Cauliflower, Sautéed Spinach	1 Protein
	(4 ounces boneless, skinless chicken breast, cut into strips, sautéed with 2 tablespoons chopped onion; 1 tablespoon sliced olives; 2 tablespoons fat-free Ital-ian dressing; ⅓ tablespoon dried basil; 1 teaspoon dried oregano; and ½ fresh plum tomato, cut into chunks)	2½ Vegetables
		2¼ Fats
	Steamed cauliflower (½ cup cauliflower florets, steamed)	
	Sautéed spinach (2 cups fresh or frozen spinach sautéed in 1⅓ tablespoons extra virgin olive oil and ¼ teaspoon each salt and ground black pepper)	
	20 ounces lemon water	
Evening Snack	20 ounces lemon water	
	Total for the Day	4 Proteins
		6 Vegetables
		2 Dairy
		3 Fats

Day 3

MEAL OR SNACK	FOODS	F-15 SERVINGS
Breakfast	Peanut Butter Smoothie (1 cup 1% milk, 1 tablespoon peanut butter, ⅓ cup whey-based protein powder, and 3 ice cubes) 1 cup green tea 20 ounces lemon water	1 Protein 1 Dairy ½ Fat
Morning Snack	1 serving **Smoked Trout and Cottage Cheese Sliders** (page 114) 20 ounces lemon water	1 Protein 1 Vegetable 1 Dairy
Lunch	Spinach Salad with Tuna (2 cups fresh spinach, 1 ounce canned artichokes, ½ cup chopped tomatoes, ½ cup sliced mushrooms, and 1 chopped hard-cooked egg tossed with 1 table-spoon white balsamic vinegar and ½ tablespoon extra virgin olive oil and topped with 3 ounces drained canned water-packed tuna) 20 ounces lemon water	1 Protein 2 Vegetables ½ Fat
Afternoon Snack	Crudités with Pine Nut Hummus (½ cup baby carrots, ½ cup cherry tomatoes, and 2 tablespoons Sabra Roasted Pine Nut Hummus) 20 ounces lemon water	1 Vegetable 1 Fat
Dinner	Stir-Fried Chicken and Vegetables over Spaghetti Squash (4 ounces boneless, skinless chicken breast, cut into strips; ¾ cup broccoli florets; 3 tablespoons chopped onion; 1 teaspoon dried rosemary; ¼ cup sliced mush-rooms; and 1 teaspoon dried thyme stir-fried in 1 table-spoon extra virgin olive oil and served over ⅓ cup cooked spaghetti squash) 20 ounces lemon water	1 Protein 2 Vegetables 1 Fat
Evening Snack	20 ounces mint lemon water	
	Total for the Day	4 Proteins 6 Vegetables 2 Dairy 3 Fats

Day 4

MEAL OR SNACK	FOODS	F-15 SERVINGS
Breakfast	Veggie Black Bean Breakfast Bowl	2 Proteins
	(4 tablespoons drained canned black beans; ½ cup chopped cauliflower florets; 1 cup fresh spinach; ½ cup chopped tomatoes; 1 clove garlic, chopped; 1 tablespoon chopped onion; 1 tablespoon chopped scallion; ½ tablespoon chopped fresh basil; and ½ tablespoon fresh thyme sautéed in ½ tablespoon extra virgin olive oil and then scrambled with 1 egg and 2 egg whites and topped with ¼ avocado, sliced)	2½ Vegetables 1 Dairy 1 Fat
	1 cup 1% milk	
	1 cup green tea	
	20 ounces lemon water	
Morning Snack	20 ounces mint lemon water	
Lunch	Shrimp Power Veggie Salad	1 Protein
	(4.5 ounces cooked shrimp, 1 cup mixed greens, ¼ cup fresh basil, ½ cup broccoli florets, and ½ cup cherry tomatoes tossed with 1 teaspoon mustard, 1 tablespoon extra virgin olive oil, and 2 tablespoons balsamic vinegar)	1½ Vegetables 1 Fat
	20 ounces lemon water	
Afternoon Snack	Cottage Cheese with Sun-Dried Tomatoes	½ Vegetable
	(½ cup 1% cottage cheese and ½ cup chopped sun-dried tomatoes)	1 Dairy
	20 ounces lemon water	
Dinner	Baked Fish with Sautéed Veggies	1 Protein
	Baked fish (dust 4 ounces of haddock with garlic powder, top with a squeeze of juice from 3 lemon wedges and 1 teaspoons trans fat–free buttery spread, and bake)	1½ Vegetables 1 Fat
	Sautéed veggies (1 tablespoon chopped onion, ½ cup chopped zucchini, ½ cup chopped Italian tomatoes, 1 teaspoon chopped fresh thyme, and ¼ cup chopped fresh basil sautéed in ⅔ tablespoon extra virgin olive oil)	
	Tossed Salad (1 cup mixed greens tossed with 1 table-spoon fat-free Italian dressing)	
	20 ounces lemon water	
Evening Snack	20 ounces mint lemon water	
Total for the Day		4 Proteins 6 Vegetables 2 Dairy 3 Fats

Day 5

MEAL OR SNACK	FOODS	F-15 SERVINGS
Breakfast	1 serving **Tuscan Breakfast Salad with Canadian Bacon** (page 108) 1 cup green tea 16 ounces lemon water	2 Proteins 1½ Vegetables 1 Fat
Morning Snack	Spiced Cottage Cheese Logs (3 stalks celery spread with ½ cup 1% cottage cheese mixed with ¼ teaspoon chili powder) 20 ounces lemon water	½ Vegetable 1 Dairy
Lunch	Chicken Salad on a Bed of Mixed Greens (3 ounces cooked boneless, skinless chicken breast, cut into chunks, mixed with 1 stalk celery, diced; 3 tablespoons chopped onion; ¼ cup chopped bell pepper; 1 tablespoon coconut oil; and 1 tablespoon lemon juice, served over 1 cup mixed greens and ½ cup chopped baby kale and topped with ¼ teaspoon paprika and ¼ teaspoon ground black pepper) 20 ounces lemon water	1 Protein 2 Vegetables 1 Fat
Afternoon Snack	Turkey Lettuce Wraps (1 ounce roast turkey breast and 2 teaspoons mustard divided and wrapped in 2 leaves butterhead or leaf lettuce) 1 cup 1% milk 20 ounces lemon water	1 Dairy
Dinner	Garlic-Rosemary Salmon with Sautéed Zucchini and Mushrooms Garlic-rosemary salmon (top 3 ounces salmon with 3 teaspoons minced garlic, ⅛ teaspoon each salt and ground black pepper, squeeze of lemon juice from 3 lemon wedges, 2 tablespoons fresh rosemary, and ½ tablespoon extra virgin olive oil and broil) Sautéed zucchini and mushrooms (½ cup sliced zucchini, ½ cup sliced mushrooms, and 1 tablespoon chopped onion sautéed in ½ tablespoon extra virgin olive oil) Tossed Salad (2 cups mixed greens tossed with 2 tablespoons fat-free Italian dressing) 20 ounces lemon water	1 Protein 2 Vegetables 1 Fat
Evening Snack	20 ounces mint lemon water	
	Total for the Day	4 Proteins 6 Vegetables 2 Dairy 3 Fats

Day 6

MEAL OR SNACK	FOODS	F-15 SERVINGS
Breakfast	Cinnamon- and Nut-Topped Yogurt	1 Protein
	(1 container [5.3 ounces] nonfat Greek yogurt mixed with ¼ teaspoon ground cinnamon and ¼ teaspoon chopped walnuts)	2 Dairy
	1 hard-cooked egg	
	1 cup 1% milk	
	16 ounces lemon water	
	1 cup green tea	
Morning Snack	Guacamole and Crudités	1 Vegetable
	Guacamole (¼ cup pureed avocado; 1 clove garlic, minced; and ½ ounce lemon juice)	1 Fat
	Crudités (½ cup carrots; 1 stalk celery, cut into thirds; and ½ cup sliced radishes)	
	20 ounces lemon water	
Lunch	Tossed Salad with Tuna	1 Protein
	(4 ounces drained canned water-packed tuna and 2 cups mixed greens tossed with 1 tablespoon toasted sesame oil and 1 tablespoon white balsamic vinegar)	1 Vegetable
		1 Fat
	20 ounces lemon water	
Afternoon Snack	Turkey Lettuce Wraps	1 Protein
	(3 ounces roast turkey breast, ½ cup chopped fresh spinach, and 2 teaspoons mustard divided and wrapped in 4 leaves butterhead or leaf lettuce)	1 Vegetable
	20 ounces lemon water	
Dinner	Broiled Halibut and Baked Vegetables	1 Protein
	Halibut (4 ounces halibut broiled with 1 tablespoon extra virgin olive oil, juice of ½ lemon, and ⅛ teaspoon each salt and ground black pepper)	3 Vegetables
		1 Fat
	Baked vegetables (melt 1 teaspoon trans fat–free buttery spread and mix with ½ tablespoon Worcestershire sauce and ½ teaspoon reduced-sodium soy sauce; pour sauce over 12 spears asparagus and ½ cup broccoli; bake until bright green and tender)	
	Tossed Salad (2 cups mixed greens tossed with 2 tablespoons fat-free Italian dressing)	
	20 ounces lemon water	
Evening Snack	20 ounces lemon water	
	Total for the Day	4 Proteins
		6 Vegetables
		2 Dairy
		3 Fats

Day 7

MEAL OR SNACK	FOODS	F-15 SERVINGS
Breakfast	Poached Salmon with Spinach	1 Protein
	(3 ounces wild salmon fillet, poached, and 2 cups fresh spinach, steamed)	1 Vegetable
	1 cup green tea	
	20 ounces lemon water	
Morning Snack	Egg Whites with Swiss Chard and Avocado	1 Protein
	(2 cups raw Swiss chard, or baby kale if you are prone to kidney or gallstones, topped with 3 hard-cooked egg whites; ¼ avocado, sliced; and the juice of 3 lemon wedges)	1 Vegetable
		1 Dairy
		1 Fat
	1 cup 1% milk	
	20 ounces lemon water	
Lunch	California Salad	1 Protein
	(2 cups mixed greens and 3 ounces roast turkey breast tossed with 2 tablespoons fat-free Italian dressing and topped with ¼ cup pureed avocado)	1 Vegetable
		1 Fat
	20 ounces lemon water	
Afternoon Snack	Herbed Cottage Cheese	1 Dairy
	(4 ounces 1% cottage cheese mixed with 2 tablespoons chopped fresh basil)	
	20 ounces lemon water	
Dinner	Fish with Sautéed Veggies	1 Protein
	Fish (5 ounces orange roughy, broiled or grilled)	3 Vegetables
	Sautéed veggies (12 spears asparagus, ½ cup cauliflower florets, 1 tablespoon ground oregano, 3 tablespoons chopped onion, and ½ cup cherry tomatoes sautéed in 1 tablespoon extra virgin olive oil)	1 Fat
	Tossed Salad (2 cups mixed greens tossed with 2 tablespoons fat-free Italian dressing)	
	1 cup chamomile tea	
	20 ounces lemon water	
Evening Snack	20 ounces basil lemon water	
	Total for the Day	4 Proteins
		6 Vegetables
		2 Dairy
		3 Fats

Day 8

MEAL OR SNACK	FOODS	F-15 SERVINGS
Breakfast	Spinach Omelet	2 Proteins
	(½ cup fresh or frozen spinach and 1 slice [1 ounce] crumbled low-fat cheddar cheese folded into 1 medium egg and 3 egg whites, beaten together, and cooked in 1 tablespoon coconut oil and then topped with ¼ tomato, chopped)	½ Vegetable
		1 Dairy
		1 Fat
	1 Aidells Organic Chicken and Apple Sausage, broiled or grilled	
	20 ounces lemon water	
Morning Snack	20 ounces lemon water	
Lunch	Tossed Salad with Roast Turkey Breast	1 Protein
	(3 ounces roast turkey breast, ½ cup cucumber slices, 2 cups mixed greens, and ½ cup cherry tomatoes tossed with 2 tablespoons fat-free Italian dressing)	1½ Vegetables
	20 ounces lemon water	
Afternoon Snack	Cottage Cheese with Cucumber Sliders	1 Vegetable
	(½ cup 1% cottage cheese mixed with ¼ teaspoon chopped fresh dill and spread on 1 cup cucumber slices)	1 Dairy
	20 ounces lemon water	
Dinner	Grilled Steak with Mushrooms and Onions	1 Protein
	(4 ounces lean short-loin porterhouse steak, fat removed, cooked with 3 teaspoons trans fat–free buttery spread mixed with 1 teaspoon chopped fresh thyme and 1 teaspoon chopped fresh basil; ¾ cup sliced mushrooms; ¼ cup sliced onion; 1 clove garlic, crushed; and ⅛ teaspoon each salt and ground black pepper)	3 Vegetables
		2 Fats
	2 cups steamed green beans	
	Tossed Salad (2 cups mixed greens tossed with 1 tablespoon extra virgin olive oil and 2 tablespoons white balsamic vinegar)	
	1 cup chamomile tea	
	20 ounces lemon water	
Evening Snack	1 cup chamomile tea	
	20 ounces lemon water	
	Total for Day	4 Proteins
		6 Vegetables
		2 Dairy
		3 Fats

Grocery List, Phase 1

PANTRY ITEMS AND STAPLES (FOR ALL WEEKS, ALL PHASES)

Almond extract

Almond butter (Barney Butter, crunchy or smooth)

Almonds, raw

Amazing Grass Organic Wheat Grass Powder

Balsamic vinegar

Beef broth, fat-free, low-sodium

Black bean spaghetti (Explore Asian; available at Whole Foods and online at explore-asian.com and amazon.com)

Black rice (Nature's Earthly Choice)

Canned artichokes

Canned bamboo shoots

Canned black beans

Canned capers

Canned olives

Canned tuna, packed in water

Chamomile tea

Chicken broth, fat-free, low-sodium

Chili powder

Classico Sun-Dried Tomato Pesto

Coconut milk (unsweetened)

Coconut oil

Cornstarch

Curry powder

Dried basil

Dried oregano

Dried rosemary

Dried thyme

Eggs

Ezekiel 4:9 sprouted 100% whole grain bread

Ezekiel sprouted grain cinnamon raisin bread

Fat-free Italian dressing

Flaxseeds (ground)

Fresh basil (bunch)

Fresh dill (bunch)

Fresh mint

Fresh thyme

Garlic powder

Grated Parmesan cheese

Green tea bags

Ground black pepper

Ground cinnamon

Ground coriander

Hemp protein concentrate (Manitoba Harvest Hemp Pro 70)

Hummus

Kalamata olives

Lentils

Matcha green tea powder (Teavana brand available online at teavana.com and amazon.com)

Mayonnaise (reduced fat, made with olive oil)

Milk (1%)

Mustard (Dijon)

Olive oil (cold pressed, extra virgin)

Olive oil cooking spray (Pam)

Paprika

Peanut butter

Pecans (unsalted)

Pumpkin seeds (unsalted)

Red curry paste, Thai brand

Red quinoa (Nature's Earthly Choice)

Red wine vinegar

Sabra Roasted Pine Nut Hummus

Sabra Roasted Red Pepper Hummus

Salt

Sesame oil (toasted, pure)

Sesame seeds

Soy sauce (reduced sodium)

Sriracha chili sauce

Stewed tomatoes

Teriyaki marinade, reduced sodium

Thai chili garlic paste

Trans fat–free buttery spread

Vanilla extract

Walnuts

Whey protein concentrate

White balsamic vinegar (Alessi)

White table wine

Worcestershire sauce

PHASE I, WEEK I

MEATS AND FISH

Aidells Organic Chicken and Apple Sausage: 1 package (refrigerate or freeze unused sausages for future weeks)

Aidells Organic Sun-Dried Tomato Sausage: 1 package (refrigerate or freeze unused sausages for future weeks)

Boneless, skinless chicken breasts: 1 pound

Canadian bacon, extra lean: ¼ pound

Canned tuna, packed in water: 6 ounces

Cod: ½ pound

Haddock: ½ pound (or 1 pound if substituting halibut)

Halibut: ½ pound

Lean turkey salami: 4–6 ounces

Prosciutto di Parma: 1 package (4 ounces)

Roast turkey breast (sliced): ½ pound

Salmon: ½ pound

Shrimp: ½ pound

Trout: ¼ pound

Tuna (yellowfin): ¼ pound

DAIRY

Cheddar or Colby cheese (low fat): 1 ounce

Cottage cheese (1%): 2¼ cups

Greek yogurt (organic, nonfat, plain): 2 containers (5.3 ounces each)

Mozzarella cheese (part-skim, reduced fat) shredded: 1 ounce

Provolone cheese (reduced fat): 1 ounce

The Laughing Cow spreadable cheese: 1 box

Yogurt (organic, low fat, plain): 1 container (4 ounces)

FRUITS AND VEGETABLES

Asparagus: 1 pound

Avocado: 1

Baby carrots: 1 cup

Bell pepper: 1

Broccoli: ½ pound

Butterhead lettuce: 1 head

Carrots: 2

Cauliflower: 1 small head

Celery: 1 bag

Cucumbers: 2

Fresh spinach: 2 large bunches or 2 bags (5 ounces each)

Garlic: 2 heads

Green leaf lettuce: 1 head

Kale: ½–1 pound

Lemons: 10

Mixed greens: 14 cups

Mushrooms: 2 cups

Onions: 2

Radishes: 5

Scallions: 3

Spaghetti squash: 1

Tomatoes (cherry): 4½ cups

Tomatoes (Italian or plum): 6

Zucchini: 2

PHASE I, WEEK 2

MEATS AND FISH

Aidells Organic Chicken and Apple Sausage: 1 package (or use the previously bought package)

Boneless, skinless chicken breast: ¾ pound

Canadian bacon, extra lean: ¼ pound

Canned tuna, packed in water: 6 ounces

Cod: ½ pound

Haddock: ¼ pound

Halibut: ¼ pound

Lean short-loin porterhouse steak: ¼ pound

Lean turkey salami: ½ pound (refrigerate excess for future use)

Orange roughy: ½ pound

Roast turkey breast (sliced): ¾ pound

Salmon: ½ pound

Shrimp: ¼ pound

Trout, smoked: ¼ pound

DAIRY

Cheddar or Colby cheese (low fat): 1 ounce

Provolone cheese (reduced fat): 2 ounces

Cottage cheese (1%): 5 cups

Greek yogurt (organic, nonfat, plain): 1 container (5.3 ounces)

The Laughing Cow spreadable cheese: 1 box

Yogurt (organic, low fat, plain): 1 container (4 ounces)

FRUITS AND VEGETABLES

Asparagus: 3 pounds

Avocado: 2

Baby carrots: 1 cup

Bell pepper: 1

Broccoli: 1¼ cups

Butterhead lettuce: 1 head

Carrots: 3

Cauliflower: 2 cups

Celery: 1 head

Cucumber: 3

Fresh spinach: 6½ cups

Garlic cloves: 5

Green beans: 2 cups

Kale: 3½ cups

Lemons: 10

Lettuce leaves: 4

Mixed greens: 1½ pounds

Mushrooms: 2½ cups

Onions: 3

Radishes: 4

Scallions: 3

Spaghetti squash: 1

Swiss chard: 1 cup

Tomatoes (cherry): 4½ cups

Tomatoes (Italian or plum): 6

Zucchini: 2

The Phase 1 Recipes

To help you stay on track with this first phase of the F-15 Plan, I've created tasty recipes for delicious, filling foods that fit perfectly into this phase.

TUSCAN BREAKFAST SALAD WITH CANADIAN BACON

SERVES 1

2 ounces extra-lean Canadian bacon

1 tablespoon toasted sesame oil

2 tablespoons white balsamic vinegar

2 cups chopped lacinato kale

1 cup cherry tomatoes, halved

1 hard-cooked or 7-minute egg, halved

1. In a nonstick skillet coated with cooking spray over medium-high heat, cook the bacon for 3 to 4 minutes, or until done and slightly browned on both sides. Slice the bacon.

2. In a small bowl, whisk together the oil and vinegar.

3. Toss the kale and tomatoes in the oil and vinegar dressing.

4. Top with the egg and bacon slices and serve.

F-15 SERVINGS:	
2	Proteins
3	Vegetables
1	Fat

NUTRITION INFORMATION:	
Calories:	447
Fat:	27 g
Carbs:	32 g
Protein:	30 g

BLACK BEAN BREAKFAST BOWL

SERVES 1

½ tablespoon extra virgin olive oil

1 tablespoon chopped onion

1 cup chopped cauliflower

1 cup fresh spinach

½ cup chopped tomatoes

1 tablespoon chopped scallion

1 teaspoon fresh thyme

2 tablespoons chopped fresh basil

4 tablespoons drained canned black beans

1 egg, whisked

Salt and ground black pepper to taste

⅛ cup cubed avocado

1. In a medium skillet over medium heat, warm the oil. Cook the onion, cauliflower, spinach, tomatoes, scallion, thyme, and basil, stirring frequently, for about 7 minutes, or until tender but firm.

2. Add the beans and then push the bean and veggie mixture to the side of the skillet.

3. With the mixture in the skillet, remove the skillet from the heat and coat with cooking spray. Return to the heat. Add the egg and scramble, cooking for 4 to 5 minutes, or until done. Add the salt and pepper.

4. Combine the egg with the vegetables and beans. Top with the avocado and serve.

F-15 SERVINGS:

1	Protein
2½	Vegetables
1	Fat

NUTRITION INFORMATION:

Calories:	367
Fat:	16 g
Carbs:	48 g
Protein:	20 g

PROSCIUTTO BREAKFAST SALAD

SERVES 1

1 egg

1 tablespoon toasted sesame oil

2 tablespoons white balsamic vinegar

2 cups mixed greens

¼ cup fresh basil leaves

1 slice prosciutto di Parma, fat removed and torn into strips

2 tablespoons sliced red onion

1 Italian tomato, thinly sliced

Cracked black pepper to taste

1. In a small nonstick skillet coated with vegetable spray over medium heat, cook the egg for a few minutes, or until the white is set and the edges are slightly browned and the yolk is firm but not completely hardened (it will run slightly when pierced).

2. With a wire whisk or fork, whisk together the oil and vinegar until blended and smooth, about a minute or less.

3. Toss the greens, basil, prosciutto, onion, and tomato in the oil and vinegar dressing.

4. Arrange the salad on a plate and add the egg on top slightly askew.

5. Sprinkle with the pepper.

F-15 SERVINGS:

2	Proteins
2	Vegetables
1	Fat

NUTRITION INFORMATION:

Calories:	257
Fat:	17 g
Carbs:	28 g
Protein:	6 g

ZUCCHINI PIZZA WEDGES

SERVES 1

1 zucchini, cut on the diagonal into 1"-thick slices

1 ounce reduced-fat shredded mozzarella cheese

1 Aidells Organic Sun-Dried Tomato Sausage, crumbled

5 cherry tomatoes, chopped

5 leaves fresh basil, torn

1. Preheat the oven on broil setting. Coat a baking pan with cooking spray.

2. Place the zucchini on the baking pan. Top with the cheese, sausage, and tomatoes.

3. Broil for 15 minutes, or until the sausage is fully cooked and the cheese is melted and bubbly.

4. Top with the basil and serve.

F-15 SERVINGS:

1	Protein
1	Vegetable
1	Dairy

NUTRITION INFORMATION:

Calories:	270
Fat:	14 g
Carbs:	13 g
Protein:	23 g

LUNCHTIME TURKEY ROLLS

SERVES 1

½ teaspoon extra virgin olive oil

1 tablespoon red wine vinegar

¼ teaspoon dried oregano

2 ounces roast turkey breast, cut into bite-size strips

1 serving lean turkey salami, cut into bite-size strips

1 slice (1 ounce) reduced-fat provolone cheese, cut into bite-size strips

¼ cup sliced white mushrooms

⅛ cup chopped bell pepper

⅛ cup red onion slices

4 leaves butterhead lettuce

1. In a small bowl, combine the oil, vinegar, and oregano. Add the turkey, salami, cheese, mushrooms, pepper, and onion. Toss to mix well.

2. Scoop the turkey mixture into the lettuce leaves, roll, and serve. If desired, secure with toothpicks.

Note: If packing for the next day's lunch, roll the lettuce leaves in damp paper towels and place in a resealable plastic bag, and spoon the turkey mixture into an airtight container. Refrigerate overnight (or for up to 3 days for the turkey mixture). To bring to work, pack in an insulated lunch box with an ice pack.

F-15 SERVINGS:	
1	Protein
1	Vegetable
1	Dairy

NUTRITION INFORMATION:	
Calories:	238
Fat:	10 g
Carbs:	6 g
Protein:	29 g

15-MINUTE FISH WITH CUCUMBER SAUCE

SERVES 1

3 ounces haddock

¼ teaspoon salt

¼ teaspoon ground pepper

¼ teaspoon garlic powder

¼ cup peeled and chopped cucumber

⅓ cup chopped fresh dill, divided

1 ounce low-fat plain yogurt

2 teaspoons mustard

½ tablespoon reduced-fat olive oil mayonnaise

3 lemon wedges, divided

1. Season the fish with the salt, pepper, and garlic powder.

2. Place the fish on a microwaveable dish and cover with vented clear plastic wrap. Microwave on high power for 4 to 7 minutes, or until the fish flakes with a fork.

3. While the fish is cooking, mix the cucumber, most of the dill, the yogurt, mustard, mayonnaise, and juice from 1 lemon wedge. Blend well.

4. Drizzle the cucumber sauce over the cooked fish. Garnish with the remaining lemon wedges and dill.

F-15 SERVINGS:

1	Protein
¼	Vegetable
½	Fat

NUTRITION INFORMATION:

Calories:	121
Fat:	4 g
Carbs:	5 g
Protein:	16 g

SMOKED TROUT AND COTTAGE CHEESE SLIDERS

SERVES 1

2 ounces smoked trout, cut into bite-size pieces

½ cup 1% cottage cheese

⅛ cup finely chopped fresh dill

1 tablespoon lemon juice

1 cup cucumber slices (1"–2" thick)

Thin lemon slices for garnish

1–2 small sprigs fresh dill for garnish

1. In a shallow bowl, add the trout, cottage cheese, dill, and lemon juice. Mix well into a spreadable consistency.

2. Spread the trout mixture onto the cucumber slices. Top each with a slice of lemon and a sprig of dill.

F-15 SERVINGS:

1	Protein
1	Vegetable
1	Dairy

NUTRITION INFORMATION:

Calories:	228
Fat:	7 g
Carbs:	9 g
Protein:	29 g

15-MINUTE SPAGHETTI SQUASH

SERVES 4

1 spaghetti squash (about 2½ pounds), halved lengthwise and seeds removed

2 teaspoons margarine, melted

1 teaspoon white wine Worcestershire sauce or Worcestershire sauce

½ teaspoon dried dillweed

Dash of ground black pepper

1. In a shallow baking dish, place one squash half cut side down (reserve the other half for another use). Microwave, uncovered, on high power for 10 to 14 minutes, half-turning the dish twice, or until the pulp can just be pierced with a fork.

2. Meanwhile, combine the margarine, Worcestershire sauce, dillweed, and pepper.

3. Shred and separate the squash pulp into strands with a fork. Rake the squash from the shell and place in a serving dish. Toss with the margarine mixture.

F-15 SERVINGS:

1	Vegetable

NUTRITION INFORMATION (PER SERVING):

Calories:	52
Fat:	2 g
Carbs:	7 g
Protein:	1 g

CHICKEN WITH TOMATOES AND OLIVES

SERVES 1

4 ounces boneless, skinless chicken breast

¼ teaspoon ground black pepper

¼ cup cherry tomatoes

1½ tablespoons oil and vinegar dressing, divided

5 large kalamata olives, chopped

2 tablespoons crumbled feta cheese

⅛ cup fresh basil leaves, torn

1. Coat a nonstick grill pan with cooking spray. Preheat over medium-high heat.

2. Sprinkle the chicken evenly with the pepper. Grill the chicken for 6 minutes on each side, or until a thermometer inserted in the thickest portion registers 165°F. Keep warm.

3. In a medium skillet over medium heat, cook the tomatoes, half of the dressing, and the olives, stirring occasionally, for 2 minutes, or until the tomatoes are slightly softened and the mixture is thoroughly heated.

4. Brush the chicken with the remaining dressing and cut into ¾" slices.

5. Top the chicken slices with the tomato mixture and sprinkle with the cheese. Garnish with the basil leaves.

F-15 SERVINGS:

1	Protein
¼	Vegetable
1½	Fat

NUTRITION INFORMATION:

Calories:	312
Fat:	20 g
Carbs:	2 g
Protein:	29 g

So Many Reasons to Move

Exercise is an important part of weight loss, weight maintenance, and the F-15 Plan. But listen, I know it can be hard to jump into an exercise regimen, especially if you haven't exercised much (or at all) in the past. That's why I make it easy to get started with my 15-Minute Moves. These quick exercise routines can be done whenever you have 15 minutes to spare. Because they're fast and easy, they can fit into even the busiest schedule.

You may have heard news reports lately that suggest exercise doesn't help much with weight loss. It's true that exercise alone can't burn up enough calories to bring about weight loss for most people. After all, you can wipe out an hour on the treadmill with a couple of cookies. But after working with thousands of people over the years, I can tell you that success is much more likely when you combine diet changes and exercise. It's not just about calorie burn. Exercise revs up your metabolism and gives you energy. Plus, it delivers numerous health benefits that go above and beyond weight loss. Don't listen to the people who tell you exercise isn't necessary. I believe that it absolutely is!

If you need more convincing, then chew on this: Research has found that people who maintain weight loss long-term are taking exercise seriously. The National Weight Control Registry tracks the habits of thousands of people who have successfully lost weight. Registry members have lost an average of 66 pounds and have kept it off for 5.5 years. Of those in the registry, more than 90 percent exercise for an average of 1 hour a day. That may sound like a lot, but once you start working exercise into your life, it's easier than you may think to accumulate an hour of activity. Many of the people in the registry started with just 15 minutes a day and worked up from there.

Experts recommend 30 minutes of moderate exercise per day, most days of the week. Even more than that is great for weight loss. But don't worry—you don't have to start out by exercising for half an hour a day every day. Instead, start with my 15-Minute Moves. Once you build a daily 15-minute exercise habit, start adding more exercise into your life. Even if you're obese, you can start exercising (as long as your doctor says it's okay). You don't have to begin by running for an hour or going to a difficult exercise class. Just take a walk! Even if you can walk slowly for only 5 minutes, that's a start—and before you know it, you'll be able to walk longer and faster.

You may be wondering why I'm so hopped up on exercise. You may think it's enough just to eat less, and you may be thinking, why do I have to bother with exercise? The truth is, you can lose weight without exercising. But it's a whole lot better for your body and your health to get out there and move.

So, why should you exercise? I'll tell you why—here are eight great reasons.

REASON #I: EXERCISE LOWERS DISEASE RISK

Studies have found that if you exercise, you reduce your risk of developing certain diseases *even if you don't lose weight*. That's right—even if you start exercising and don't lose a single pound, your risk of some diseases goes down. But get this: If you exercise and lose weight, you're in an even better position to lower your risk of diseases such as heart disease, stroke, diabetes, some forms of cancer, age-related dementia, depression, and arthritis, to name a few. Exercise helps to lower blood pressure, raises HDL ("healthy") cholesterol, lowers LDL ("lousy") cholesterol and triglycerides, and helps keep blood sugar stable. If there were a pill as effective as exercise, every doctor in America would be prescribing it to all of their patients.

REASON #2: EXERCISE BOOSTS WEIGHT LOSS

People argue a lot about whether diet or exercise is better for weight loss. The fact is that unless you're exercising for hours a day, exercise alone won't bring about amazing weight loss. You have to cut back on servings and portion sizes, like with the F-15 Plan. Furthermore, you have to put the right foods in your body in the proper quantities. Yes, abs are made in the kitchen, but exercise really does do a body good! And exercise definitely boosts weight-loss success. Not only do you burn calories while you're exercising, but you rev up your metabolism in a way that benefits you for several hours afterward. That's right—when you exercise, you continue to burn extra calories even at rest. So if you go back to work and sit at your desk after you work out, you're continuing to burn more calories while you sit than you would if you hadn't exercised.

Exercise boosts weight loss for another reason, as well. I call it the virtue factor. When we exercise, we feel so great about ourselves that it's much easier afterward to say no to food temptations. When you come in from a long walk or an invigorating swim, you're not going to sit down and have a big bag of potato chips, right? You're going to feel so virtuous that you'll be perfectly happy with a plate of vegetables for a snack. This helps bring about weight loss.

Finally, when you exercise, you build muscle, and maintaining muscle mass burns more calories than maintaining fat. That's right—if you have extra muscle, you burn more calories just sitting still than you do when you have less muscle. Over time, simply having more muscle actually leads to better weight loss. You can't beat that!

REASON #3: EXERCISE IS AN AMAZING STRESS BUSTER

As I'll explain later in this chapter, chronic stress can prevent weight loss. One of the many ways to reduce the effect of stress on your body is to exercise. Walking, jogging, swimming, taking an exercise class, strength training—these activities all lead to lower levels of stress hormones in your body, which in turn helps you lose weight more successfully.

REASON #4: EXERCISE ENERGIZES YOU

It seems that something that uses energy would make you feel less energetic. But with exercise, the opposite is true: Exercise actually makes you feel more energetic. That's because it improves your muscle tone and builds endurance. When you exercise, you improve the strength of your heart and lungs, and over time, you can do more without feeling tired or out of breath. Keep on exercising, and eventually the movements that left you winded—shoveling snow, raking leaves, or chasing children or grandchildren—become easier.

REASON #5: EXERCISE STRENGTHENS BONES AND MUSCLES

When you exercise, your muscles and bones become stronger. This is important because having strong bones and muscles reduces your chances of hip fractures, falls, and osteoporosis, a disease in which bones become thin and brittle.

REASON #6: EXERCISE HELPS YOU SLEEP

Studies show that people who engage in moderate exercise sleep better than those who don't. They fall asleep more quickly and sleep more deeply. For some people, exercising too close to bedtime can keep them awake, but others find that a walk before bed is a relaxing routine. Experiment with exercise schedules to see what works best for you. Some people love an early-morning workout; others prefer to exercise later in the day.

REASON #7: EXERCISE CAN HELP YOU LIVE LONGER

Researchers have found that regular exercise helps lower your chances of dying early because of diseases such as heart disease, complications from diabetes, and some kinds of cancer. For example, according to the Centers for Disease Control and Prevention (CDC), people who are physically active for about 7 hours a week have a 40 percent lower risk of dying early than those who are active for less than 30 minutes a week. That's a big difference! You don't have to do large amounts of physical activity or vigorous-intensity activity to reduce your risk of premature death, according to the CDC. You can put yourself at lower risk of dying early by doing at least 150 minutes a week of moderate-intensity aerobic activity. That's just 30 minutes a day 5 days a week.

REASON #8: EXERCISE IS FUN!

If you've never exercised before, you may have rolled your eyes when you read that reason. But it's true: Once you get into it, exercise really is fun! If you don't believe me, go take a look at a spin class at a local gym or a Zumba class at your local YMCA. I also recommend that you try the Kukuwa Fitness African Dance Workout videos or class, developed by Kukuwa, a fitness pro from Ghana. The workout is high energy and effective and a super fun way to burn fat and calories. Kukuwa herself is an enormous inspiration and ball of fire! It's possible to burn up to 1,000 calories in one 60-minute workout. Find her classes and videos online at kukuwafitness.com.

I recently rediscovered spin class and found that I love it! If you do check out a spin class while you're visiting the gym, ask about a new craze called POUND. It's a class that engages your core and lower body (gluteal and quadriceps) muscles. As you perform squats and lunges, you also pound a set of drumsticks on the floor from various positions. Pounding to the beat of really dope music and building muscle at the same time can be überfun and exhilarating!

If you're a social butterfly, you might try inviting a few friends to go for a Saturday morning walk. Getting together with friends—or even strangers who share an interest in fitness—can be a load of fun. Researchers have found that exercise can boost mood; when you exercise, your brain releases feel-good neurochemicals that can go a long way toward improving your mood.

Now that you fully understand why exercise is such an important part of the F-15 Plan, here are some of my favorite 15-Minute Moves. These mini-workouts will help move you toward your weight and health goals by revving up your metabolism, building muscle, and burning fat fast. Do one a day, two a day, or more; whatever you can fit into your schedule.

Your 15-Minute Moves for Phase 1

These F-15 workouts take just 15 minutes to complete. The recommended goal for exercise is at least 30 minutes a day, most days of the week. But this can be overwhelming if you're just getting started. So, here's my advice: Start small by doing one 15-minute session per day. As you become fitter, you'll start enjoying your workouts and feeling stronger and healthier. You'll want to add in more exercise then—either additional 15-Minute Moves or other exercise, such as walking, jogging, swimming, dancing, cycling, whatever you like.

Here are a few things to keep in mind before you start.

Begin by warming up. Start your workout with a brisk 5-minute walk that increases your bloodflow and warms up your muscles. Incorporate walking knees to chest, walking hamstring curls, walking arm circles forward and backward, and lunges with rotation.

End with light stretching. After your 15-Minute Move, do some light stretching.

Check in with your doctor. Before beginning any exercise or diet plan, get your doctor's okay.

Now, do your workout! Follow the descriptions, starting on page 122. Explanations of the exercises appear after the workouts. Try the workouts in this phase and subsequent phases using the Tabata, HIIT, or AMRAP method described.

YOUR WORKOUTS THREE WAYS

1. **Tabata training 20/10**—20 seconds of all-out exercise followed by 10 seconds of rest. Each Tabata is 4 minutes in duration. Tabata workouts will have three Tabatas with a 1-minute rest between each.

2. **HIIT training (high-intensity interval training)**—High-intensity exercise intervals intermingled with lower-intensity intervals of active rest.

3. **AMRAP**—As many rounds as possible of several exercises in an allotted amount of time, 15 minutes.

Tabata Workout #1

TOTAL TIME: 15 MINUTES

1. **Burpees and Situps**—20 seconds of Burpees and 10 seconds of rest; 20 seconds of Situps (beginner level: crunches) and 10 seconds of rest; repeat the sequence for 4 minutes.

REST FOR 1 MINUTE.

2. **High Knees and Plank**—20 seconds of High Knees and 10 seconds of rest; 20 seconds of Plank and 10 seconds of rest; repeat for 4 minutes.

REST FOR 1 MINUTE.

3. **Squats and Triceps Dips**—20 seconds of Squats (advanced level: jump squats) and 10 seconds of rest; 20 seconds of Triceps Dips (advanced level: plyo triceps dips) and 10 seconds of rest; repeat for 4 minutes.

STRETCH. YOU'RE DONE!

CONGRATS! YOU MADE IT! YOU'RE AWESOME!

BURPEES

My 15-Minute Moves incorporate something called burpees. No, this isn't something that happens to you when you drink a soda too quickly. Burpees are moves that work every part of your body and all major muscle groups. They dramatically increase your heart rate for maximum calorie and fat burn. Greater intensity of movement leads to a greater boost in metabolism as well as improvement of cardiovascular health.

Here's how to do a burpee.

Step 1: Begin in a standing position.

Step 2: Drop into a squat position with your hands on the floor.

Step 3: Jump by kicking your feet back with your toes pointed toward the floor, keeping your arms extended and palms on the ground.

Step 4: Immediately return your feet to a squat position.

Step 5: Jump up to a standing position and count to four.

SITUPS

ABS (CORE STRENGTH)

Step 1: Lie on your back with your knees bent and the balls of your feet and heels flat on the floor, keeping arms at your side, with palms facing the floor.

Step 2: Place your hands on opposing shoulders, crossing your arms over your chest or interlocking your hands behind your head (which gives you a central rising point).

Step 3: Gently tighten your abdominal muscles by drawing your belly button into your spine.

Step 4: Keep your heels on the floor, with toes flat to the ground as you slowly lift your head first, followed by your shoulder blades. It helps to focus your eyes on your bent knees as you make your way up to the

PHASE I: HIGH-INTENSITY FAT BURNING   123

top of the situp. Pull your body up from the floor to a 90-degree angle or to the point where your elbows are on or past your knees.

HIGH KNEES

CARDIO

Step 1: Stand erect with your feet hip-width apart, looking straight ahead. Make sure your arms are hanging at your sides.

Step 2: Bring your knees up one at a time to hip level, as though you were going to jog in place.

Step 3: Jump from one foot to the other at the same time, lifting your knees as high as you can. Your arms should follow the motion of your legs/knees. *Note:* Beginners go slower and bring your knees as high as your body is most comfortable.

Step 4: Alternate bringing your knees up to hip level for the desired time.

PLANK

CORE, CHEST, SHOULDERS, ARMS

Place forearms on the floor, keep your elbows aligned below your shoulders, and keep arms parallel to your body about shoulder-width apart. If flat palms bother your wrists, clasp your hands together.

NOTE: A plank can be done with straight arms as well.

SQUATS

LOWER BODY (GLUTEAL AND QUADRICEPS MUSCLES)

Step 1: Stand erect, looking straight ahead, with your head and shoulders back. Keep a slight arch in your lower back, your feet hip-width apart, and your arms at your sides.

Step 2: Start to lower your body by pushing your hips back as if to sit on a chair, bending your knees and pushing your body weight into your heels. Remember to keep your chest up and shoulders back while bending from your hips. Always keep a neutral spine for protection.

Step 3: Sit as low as possible (the goal is to have your legs parallel with the floor, but go as low as is comfortable for you; never exceed your comfort level). As you sit, raise your arms in front of your body or raise them over your head to assist with balance.

HIIT Workout #1

TOTAL TIME: 15 MINUTES

1. 1 minute of Burpees (beginner: 30 seconds)
2. 30 seconds of Crunches (beginner: 15 seconds)
3. Rest for 30 seconds
4. 1 minute of High Knees (beginner: 30 seconds)
5. 30 seconds of Plank (beginner: 15 seconds)
6. Rest for 30 seconds
7. 1 minute of Squats (beginner: 30 seconds)
8. 30 seconds of Triceps Dips
9. Rest for 30 seconds
10. 1 minute of Jumping Jacks
11. 30 seconds of Plank
12. Rest for 30 seconds
13. Repeat the cycle until you've reached the 15-minute mark. Go!

STRETCH. YOU'RE DONE!
CONGRATS! YOU MADE IT! YOU'RE AWESOME!

Step 4: Pause at the bottom of the motion before driving through your heels to stand. Keep your knees behind your toes and your weight in your heels for safety and to prevent injury.

NOTE: For increased calorie burn, try doing squats with a pair of dumbbells (3 to 5 pounds each). Keep the dumbbells at your sides as you squat. This works well with lunges and walking lunges, too!

TRICEPS DIPS

UPPER BODY (TRICEPS)

Step 1: Sit on the side of a bench (or a sturdy chair, bathtub, or step). Place your hands on the edge of the bench, positioning your feet away from the bench. Keep your arms straight.

Step 2: Slide your hips off the edge of the bench, and rest your heels on the floor with straight legs (bend them if you need to).

AMRAP Workout #1

TOTAL TIME: 15 MINUTES

1. **Pushups**—Do 15 reps.

2. **Alternating Lunges**—Do 15 reps on each leg.

3. **Jumping Jacks**—Do 15 reps.

4. Rest as needed between rounds. Repeat cycle, doing as many rounds as possible for 15 minutes.

STRETCH. YOU'RE DONE!

CONGRATS! YOU MADE IT! YOU'RE AWESOME!

Step 3: Lower your body as far as you can, bending your arms until you feel a slight stretch in your chest or shoulders, or until your hips touch the floor. (Kudos to you if you go that far on your first try!)

Step 4: Raise your body and repeat.

CRUNCHES

ABS AND OBLIQUES

Lie on your back with knees bent and feet flat on the floor a hop-width apart. Place your arms folded across your chest. Raise head and shoulders (upper body), squeezing abdominal muscles off the floor. Hold at the top for 3 breaths, then return to start position and repeat. You should feel tension in abdominal muscles.

PUSHUPS

UPPER BODY (TRICEPS, SHOULDERS)

Step 1: Start by lying face down with your hands on the floor shoulder-width apart, palms down. Keep your weight distributed between your hands and feet, with your toes pointed toward the floor. Prop your body up to plank position, keeping rigid and straight.

Step 2: Lower your body until your chest nears the floor at the bottom of the movement, and return to the start position (bend your knees and push up from the knee if you need help lifting your entire body). Congrats! You just did one repetition!

Step 3: Remember to move in a smooth, fluid motion using and tightening your core. At the top of the pushup, exhale as you lower you body back to the floor, and inhale as you lift off for the next rep.

BEGINNER LEVEL: Keep your knees bent to push up from your knees.

ALTERNATING LUNGES

LOWER BODY (GLUTEAL AND QUADRICEPS MUSCLES)

Step 1: From a standing position, step forward with one leg, bending both knees.

Step 2: Lower your body so that both knees are at 90-degree angles.

Step 3: Keep your chest up and your shoulders back. Make sure your core is engaged, with your front knee behind your toe.

Step 4: Push back to standing and repeat with the opposite leg.

JUMPING JACKS

CARDIO

Step 1: Standing with your feet together and your arms by your sides, jump, raising your arms above your head and bringing your palms together at the top of the movement. Then return your feet to the floor with a smooth coordinated motion.

Step 2: Return to the starting position, bringing your arms back to your side, and repeat the motion until you have completed the number of jumping jacks needed to progress to your next exercise.

BEGINNER LEVEL: Step one leg at a time out to the side while reaching your arms above your head.

Be proud of yourself! You're doing what you thought you couldn't do. Prove to yourself everyday that you can do something more. You're stronger than you think!

Stress and Weight

Let's face it: Stress is a big problem for us all. We live busy lives filled with many expectations. Our bosses want that latest project finished right away—preferably yesterday. Our kids need rides to baseball practice, help with homework, support when they're making decisions about their education. We have bills to pay, household chores to be completed, and problems to be solved. The world around us throws lots of stress our way, too, with worrisome news coming in at all hours of the day and night. Even our electronic devices stress us out, with constant interruptions from text messages, e-mails, news alerts, and everything else that comes over the digital transom.

Our minds and bodies respond to all of these stressors. When you are faced with stress, your body reacts with a physiological fight-or-flight response that is designed to prepare you either to confront or run away from what's stressing you. Your heart rate speeds up, your brain releases stress hormones, your breathing becomes more rapid, your metabolism revs up, and your blood carries extra oxygen to your muscles to prepare them for action. All of this happens instantaneously and has been fine-tuned by evolution to allow us to keep ourselves safe in the face of danger.

The stress response is fantastically useful if your stressor is a specific danger (for example, if you're about to be attacked by an angry dog, the stress response gives you the physical wherewithal to fight or flee). But if the cause of your stress is something that can't be chased away easily and that lingers in your life indefinitely—a toxic relationship, an unreasonable boss, or constant money problems—you can't run or fight. You have to deal with it over time, which causes long-term chronic stress that can last for days, weeks, or even years.

When your fight-or-flight reaction gets stuck in the on position, you suffer physically and emotionally. News flash: Weight gain happens to be one of the physical responses to the seemingly unending stressors that you experience. I mentioned that stress was a major cause of hypertension for African Americans, based on a large national study, the first of its kind, in my first book, *Dr. Ro's Ten Secrets to Livin' Healthy*. Now we know that stress not only causes high blood pressure but also weight gain. Research has shown that chronic stress contributes to weight gain, and that—get this—it's harder to lose weight when you feel stressed.

That's why I recommend stress-reduction and relaxation techniques as part of the F-15 Plan. Relaxation is the antidote to chronic stress. We can't always change what causes us stress in life. But we can change our response to it by taking steps to reduce the effects of stress on our bodies. One way to do this is by practicing stress-reduction techniques for at least 15 minutes a day.

Success Story

Amy Gidley

20 pounds lost
15.3 inches lost overall

Amy is a registered nurse who works the night shift. At times she fluctuates between the night and day shift, so this schedule wreaks havoc on her weight. She is also a mother of adult children and thought her childbearing years were over but then gave birth to a rambunctious baby boy. During her pregnancy, the only thing Amy enjoyed was eating! She downed pasta with cream and cheese sauces by the pound. She also craved potato chips and french fries like they were the Last Supper. Naturally, she gained more than the recommended 20 to 30 pounds of pregnancy weight.

Because Amy had her baby after age 40, a time when metabolism and hormones start to plummet, she found it harder to shed the excess baby weight. She came to me to help her ditch the sweet tea, sodas, french fries, and fat-filled pasta dishes. Finding time to exercise was also hard for her.

We tested Amy's hormones (using blood tests) and discovered her cortisol, thyroid hormone, estrogen, testosterone, and progesterone levels were adversely affecting her weight and sleep patterns. My medical director and I concluded that Amy would benefit from bioidentical hormone pellet therapy to stabilize her hormones and improve her weight loss.

We planned Amy's eating schedule such that if she worked from 7 p.m. to 7 a.m., she would have the bulk of her

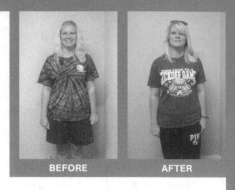

BEFORE • AFTER

calories by 6 p.m., her lighter next meal between 9 p.m. and 10 p.m., two 150- to 200-calorie snacks overnight, and then nothing except lemon water until a light breakfast between 8 a.m. and 9 a.m. the next morning. We chose go-to snacks for work: DIY protein bars, tuna pouches and mixed raw veggies, raw almonds, fresh fruit, and a trail mix made of popcorn, nuts, and seeds with a chocolate drizzle.

Amy also took on her reliance on diet sodas, which have been linked to obesity and found to trick the brain into craving sugary foods and beverages, and replaced it with lemon water. Not only did the lemon water help her kick her diet soda habit, but the squeeze of lemon added to her water increased her body's alkalinity to reduce inflammation.

And, of course, we got Amy exercising. She squeezed activity in whenever possible; for example, she took brisk 15-minute walks after the night shift to burn extra calories and rev up her metabolism.

Now Amy feels better than ever. "I wanted to lose weight to feel better and to see my son grow up. Dr. Ro's plan wasn't the easiest to do at first, but now it's second nature."

HOW RELAXATION HELPS

Relaxation techniques can be used to elicit what's known as the relaxation response. This is our own inborn capacity to reduce internal stress. Harvard researcher Dr. Herbert Benson, the father of mind-body medicine, first identified the relaxation response.

When you use relaxation techniques, you move your body toward entering a deeply relaxed state of calmness. When we become deeply relaxed, some fantastic things happen. There is a measurable reduction in blood pressure, heart rate, breathing rate, stress hormone levels in the blood, and muscle tension. We feel less anxious and more confident, better prepared to face the challenges of life.

Why is it important to make relaxation part of your weight-loss plan? And why do I recommend that you set aside at least 15 minutes each day as you work your way through the F-15 Plan? Here are a few reasons.

Stress can make us eat more. When you are stressed, your body releases a stress hormone called *cortisol*. Chronically high levels of cortisol actually increase your desire for food, making you think you're hungry even if you're not. And if you eat while you're stressed, you are much less likely to notice when your body sends signals that you're full and have eaten enough, which often leads to overeating. Studies have found that stress is associated with excess weight. No one is exactly sure how they are connected, but possible answers come from a 2016 animal study published in the journal *BBA Molecular and Cell Biology of Lipids*. The study found that chronic stress triggers the production of a protein known as betatrophin. This protein is believed to slow down fat burning. Over time, slower fat burn may lead to weight gain.

We eat to relieve stress. Eating actually can make you feel better when you're stressed. But that doesn't mean it's a good way of dealing with stress; it doesn't solve the real problem. The soothing feelings you get when you gobble up a pint of ice cream or a bag of cookies are temporary at best. They disappear soon after eating and are usually replaced with feelings of shame and guilt. Over time, being overweight causes a different kind of emotional stress—which can cause you to eat even more!

We crave carbohydrates when we're stressed. When our bodies experience the fight-or-flight response, energy moves to our muscles in order to help us confront or escape from our stressors. When this happens, insulin reactions cause us to crave carbohydrates and sweet foods, which are the quickest source of energy. Eating high-carbohydrate foods—such as breads, cakes, cookies, pasta, and all the rest—cause blood-sugar spikes that are followed by rapid drops in blood sugar. When blood sugar falls quickly, guess what happens next? You're right—you crave even *more* carbohydrates. It's a vicious cycle that leads to weight gain and raises diabetes risk.

Stress increases dangerous belly fat. Chronically high levels of stress hormones prompt your body to store fat around the midsection. Referred to as visceral fat, this belly fat is especially risky because it is linked to higher rates of diabetes and heart disease.

So, how can you prevent stress from sabotaging your weight-loss efforts? Don't worry—I've got your back. I'll provide a few stress-busting exercises you can do in just 15 minutes. Each one will help you relax and lower the impact of stress on your mind and your body. And try yoga, meditation, journaling, and other stress-reduction techniques to help you relax each day.

USING MINDFULNESS TO LOSE WEIGHT— AND GAIN HAPPINESS

So much of what we do in life is mindless. We often go through our days without paying attention to what we're thinking and feeling, or while engaged in one activity, we're thinking about another. This can lead to unhappiness, stress, and overall dissatisfaction with life. And it can lead to weight gain because it allows us to take action without really thinking, muddling through life mindlessly. We can reverse the habit of mindlessness by going in the opposite direction and cultivating a practice of mindfulness.

Let's start by defining the word *mindfulness*. It's a practice of becoming fully aware of what's going on in the present moment. When you're mindful, you're aware of everything going on around you. You become completely aware of exactly what you are thinking and feeling. Instead of standing at the kitchen counter chopping produce while thinking of the reasons you didn't respond to the person who insulted you at the grocery store, practicing mindfulness means you'd concentrate completely on the way the knife slices and dices, on cupping your fingers to prevent an accident; you'd pay attention to the bright orange color of the carrots and the juice flowing from the bright red tomatoes. In this mindful state, you'd be far less likely to cut your finger, because you'd be focused on what's before you and not wandering off in thought to someplace else in your mind.

Mindfulness is awareness; it involves paying attention to what your senses tell you about your environment—to what you see, hear, taste, smell, and feel. Practicing mindfulness means being aware of whether or not you are warm or cold, happy or sad, tired or rested, and it is void of all judgment of yourself and others.

When you're mindful, you may notice that you're feeling anxious, but you don't criticize yourself for it. If judgments arise, you let them go, focusing on simply being aware of what's going on in and around you.

Mindfulness helps you to relax because it takes you away from the thoughts, worries, regrets, and fears that constantly circulate in all of our minds at one time or another, if not constantly. When you're mindful, you stop yourself from dwelling on the past or the future and focus on the now—the only true time we really ever have, the present moment.

Practicing mindfulness means you look for things to appreciate in the here and now—the sun on your face, the wind at your back. Instead of regretting yesterday or worrying about tomorrow (which, by the way, you'll never control), you look for the little things that make you happy right this second! You can do *anything* mindfully—exercise, eat, shower, or even have sex. Yes! I said sex! It all comes down to paying attention, using your senses to appreciate the present moment, and letting go of everything else. I'm not going to show you how to have sex mindfully—you're on your own for that, my friend—but I will "walk you through" a demonstration of mindful walking. I'll also tell you about another fantastic way of relaxing, using a technique known as *prayerful meditation.*

15-MINUTE STRESS BUSTER: MINDFUL WALKING

Mindful walking is a great stress buster because you can do it anytime, anywhere. It can take you away from your stressors while providing some of the mind-body benefits of activity. A 15-minute mindful walk can refresh and energize you, and you can fit it in during any part of your day. Here's how to do it.

Choose a route. Where will you walk? The best place is somewhere beautiful—a leafy park or on a beach, for example. But let's face it: Most of us can't just run off to a park for a 15-minute walk every day. So pick the nicest spot you can get to easily, preferably outdoors—but inside is fine, too, as long as there aren't too many distractions.

Start walking. A mindful walk isn't a workout, so there's no need to be speedy. Instead, walk at a relatively slow pace. Set aside anything that might interrupt you—turn off your phone, and don't even listen to music. This is about connecting to a power greater than yourself, and it's about going deeper, being introspective to get in touch with the real you for more peace and security.

Focus on your senses. As you walk, spend a minute or two paying attention to the information that each of your senses is gathering. Start with sight: What do you see? If you're outdoors, you may see birds flying overhead or beautiful flowers blooming. Move to the rest of your senses: What do you hear, smell, taste? How does the sidewalk feel beneath your feet? Can you feel the sun on your face? Are breezes blowing through your hair?

Let go of negatives. If negative thoughts pop into your mind, let them go. Tell yourself you'll think about them later, because right now you're focusing on what your senses are experiencing right this moment. Letting go of difficult thoughts isn't always easy, but as you practice mindfulness, you'll get better and better at it.

End with a few deep breaths. At the end of 15 minutes (or longer if you need it), stop and take a few deep breaths. Thank yourself for making time to give yourself the gift of mindfulness.

Go back into the world with a fresh awareness. As you return to work, your family, or whatever other responsibilities you have, try to carry with you the mindfulness you practiced on your walk. The goal of mindfulness is to incorporate it into your entire day so you can live a more conscious, mindful life. When you're mindful, you enjoy life more and are better able to make decisions that benefit your health and that fortify your spirit.

15-MINUTE STRESS BUSTER: PRAYERFUL MEDITATION

Prayerful meditation works for people of any faith and those of no faith—provided prayer is a source of comfort to you. It works for people who may not practice any organized religion or consider themselves religious but who have a sense of connection to a spirit that joins us all. I find prayerful meditation fulfilling because it allows me to connect with God in a way that gives me peace. Meditation and prayer help me to become centered and prepared to take on the day, calmer, focused, and intentioned.

During prayerful meditation, you focus on something that brings you closer to God or whatever you may call the power greater than yourself. Some people choose to think about a word, phrase, or mantra—such as "God is good" or "the Lord is my shepherd" or "*Modeh Ani*" (I give thanks)—or some simply think about a sound, such as Ahhhhh, which in all faiths, religions, and spiritual teachings connects to the same power. It is literally the sound made when all speak of God. Once you've chosen a focal point, you're ready to try prayerful meditation. Here's how to do it.

Find a quiet space. Turn off your phone, and lower the lights if possible. Make sure the temperature is comfortable—not too warm, not too cold. If it's chilly, throw a sweater or blanket over you. If you like, play inspirational music, light candles, or burn incense, but none of that is necessary unless it's what you enjoy.

Sit in a comfortable position. Make sure you're comfortable. If you lie down, set a timer (unless you're trying to pray yourself to sleep).

Close your eyes. Or keep them open—whatever works best for you.

Breathe normally for a few breaths. Prepare yourself for meditation by breathing in through your nose and out through your mouth.

Take a few deeper breaths. Begin breathing more deeply, filling your lungs and expanding your belly as you breathe. Now, start to focus on your prayerful expression. Say it to yourself (or out loud, if you'd like) with each inhale. Then, let the memory of the thought linger in your mind as you exhale.

Visualize your peace. If you have chosen to visualize a sacred place, do that as you inhale and exhale. As you do in visualization relaxation exercises, use your senses to fully experience the place.

Continue breathing deeply. Inhale slowly to the count of five, thinking or speaking your prayerful expression, and exhale slowly to the count of five. As you inhale, imagine yourself bringing peace into your body and mind. As you exhale, imagine yourself letting go of stress and anxiety.

Don't judge if your mind wanders. Inevitably your mind will go in different directions as you practice this or any type of meditation in the beginning (you'll start thinking about what your coworker said to you that morning or the items on your grocery list). When that happens, acknowledge it and then refocus on your breathing. It's normal for your mind to wander. As you practice meditation and become more experienced with it, you will become more focused. But, whatever you do, don't judge yourself for not being "good enough" at meditation, because that defeats the whole purpose of the exercise. Experiencing those kinds of defeatist feelings can spill over in other areas of your life, and that's the opposite of what we're working to achieve here.

End your meditation gently. When you finish meditating, open your eyes slowly and take a few more deep breaths. Thank God for the peace you've received during your prayerful meditation. Stand up, stretch, and thank yourself for taking the time to practice meditating and to finally do something for you. Give yourself a big hug from me. You deserve it!

If you'd like to learn more about structured relaxation techniques, check out your local YMCA or community education programs, which may offer classes in meditation, mindfulness, or yoga. The better you become at managing stress, the more likely you are to achieve and maintain all of your life's goals, including weight loss.

In the Next Chapter: Phase 2 of the **F-15** Plan

You should be incredibly proud of yourself. You've finished one phase of the F-15 Plan, and now you have everything you need to dive into Phase 2. In the next chapter, I'll show you how you can continue to lose weight while adding in more food choices. I'll show you more great exercises you can use to rev up your metabolism and burn fat and calories. And I'll share more recipes and meal plans that will help you stay on track. Keep up the good work. You're doing great!

Chapter 5

PHASE 2: ASSIMILATION

*Each day God allows us to open our eyes
is a new opportunity to get it right. Don't beat
yourself up; use the energy to do better.*
—Dr. Ro

Congratulations! You've completed Phase 1 of the F-15 Plan, and you're now ready to move on to Phase 2. By now you should be making some great progress. Not only is your metabolism humming along at a revved-up rate, but your body is improving its ability to burn fat. You should be starting to see some exciting changes on your scale, too. Most people who follow the F-15 Plan have lost about 5 pounds by now—but keep in mind that results vary, and it's not unusual to have lost a few pounds more or less than that. Your weight loss will continue as you move from Phase 1 to Phase 2.

In Phase 1, we focused on high-intensity fat burning. Now, in Phase 2, we continue to make fat burning a priority, but we're shifting our focus a bit in order to give you more choices of delicious food. I call this the Assimilation Phase of the F-15 Plan because it makes space for your body to assimilate some of your favorite foods to enjoy! My goal is to have you eating a well-balanced diet with controlled portion sizes of health-giving foods. For example, Phase 2 includes fruit, as well as some additional vegetables that were excluded during Phase 1.

During Phase 2, you will continue to work exercise into your daily life by using my 15-Minute Moves. You can keep using the moves from Phase 1 and add in the additional move choices I offer in Phase 2.

And, of course, Phase 2 provides the menu-planning help you need, with a 15-Day Meal Plan and more super-easy, tasty recipes that you'll fall in love with and that fit perfectly into the Phase 2 guidelines.

The Phase 2 Servings Plan

Phase 2 includes many of the same great choices as Phase 1. For example, you'll continue to eat plenty of power-packed foods in each meal, including lean protein, nutrient-rich vegetables, dairy, and fats. And during this phase, you'll also start including fruit in your daily meal plans.

It's this simple: Each day during Phase 2, you'll eat a total of 15 servings of food: four servings of protein (lean meat, poultry, fish, beans, nuts, seeds, and eggs), four servings of vegetables, two servings of fruit, two servings of low-fat dairy foods, and three servings of fat.

BEHIND THE SERVINGS

As I explained in Phase 1, I've carefully thought out the serving strategy of each phase of the F-15 Plan to make it as effective and easy to follow as possible. Some of the choices in Phase 1 remain in Phase 2; others are different. Here's a quick guide to what you'll be eating in this phase.

Protein: This macronutrient—which is found in meat, poultry, fish, eggs, nuts, legumes, and seeds—continues to be a major player in the F-15 Plan. Eating protein helps to keep your metabolism going at

PHASE 2 SERVINGS

During Phase 2 of the F-15 Plan, you'll eat the following foods.

- ✓ 4 servings of protein
- ✓ 4 servings of vegetables
- ✓ 2 servings of fruit
- ✓ 2 servings of low-fat dairy
- ✓ 3 servings of fat

TOTAL: **15 servings per day**

(For a full review of serving sizes, see the tables in Chapter 3.)

Success Story

Johnjalene Woods

25 pounds lost

5.5 inches lost from the belly area

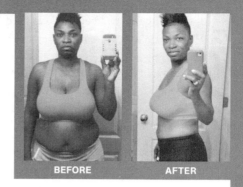

BEFORE   AFTER

Johnjalene is a crazy-busy football mama to a star athlete. She's also a hair stylist who owns a lucrative salon. When she first came to me, she was at a loss for what to do to get control of her life. She was used to yo-yo dieting and occasionally working out, but she had hit a plateau for the last time. She told me she wanted a plan that would help her not only lose her last 25 pounds but also maintain a healthy weight for the rest of her life. No problem!

Johnjalene had done practically every diet and weight-loss plan on the planet and nothing stuck. She would fall off the wagon again and again, never really making any permanent lifestyle changes. So this time we needed to help her accomplish that. She was well versed in the kinds of foods to eat, but the portions were iffy.

Johnjalene was under the impression that juicing was a weight-loss panacea. I asked her to bring in the ingredients and a recipe for her favorite juice. What we discovered was that she was consuming an extra 450 calories a day in juice alone! I know what you're thinking: But juice is a good thing, right? Not exactly. It's high in sugar and calories, and it is far inferior to whole fruit. We got rid of that version of her favorite juice first. Then we adjusted the ingredient amounts such that she could incorporate them into her daily F-15 Meal Plan, accounting for her prescribed serving sizes.

Because of her busy schedule, Johnjalene ate lunch between clients. She often ate a healthy and nutritious lunch that included vegetables, but the portions were too large, and the manner in which her vegetables were prepared also needed a reboot. When she cooked greens, she followed her upbringing and seasoned them with fatback or ham hocks. We nixed those options, and I taught her how to sauté her greens with a small amount of extra virgin olive oil, $\frac{1}{2}$ cup of water, a pinch of salt and ground red pepper, with a dash of hot-pepper sauce and a squeeze of lemon at the end. She had never had greens cooked this way and found them to be delicious!

Johnjalene also walked, but only intermittently because her schedule was so hectic. We weaved partial workouts into her daily activities. I also asked her to walk laps around her building and parking lot at work. We then added 1- or 2-pound weights to the walk and later lunges and squats during her workload at her salon. We eventually got her doing 15-minute workout routines before and sometimes after work.

Her hard work paid off. "The fact that my belly fat has melted away is a huge relief," Johnjalene says.

full-speed, helps to keep you satiated, and leads your body to lose the fat and gain muscle, as it increases overall weight loss.

Vegetables: It's important to continue making vegetables part of your daily eating plan during Phase 2. That's because veggies, which are high in fiber, help to fill you up and satiate you. And, remember, they have fewer calories, are übernutritious, and have more water than most other foods. They belong in most or all of your meals and snacks.

As you learned in Chapter 4, there are two kinds of vegetables in the F-15 Plan: Everyday Vegetables and Occasional Vegetables. In Phase 1, you had an abundance of Everyday Vegetables because they are high in fiber, nutrients, and water while being low in calories and carbohydrates. Now in Phase 2, you can have even more! In this phase you now have an additional two servings a week of Occasional Vegetables. Be sure to count them in your F-15 daily serving tally. (See Chapter 3 for a full list of vegetables.)

During Phase 2, continue to think of Everyday Vegetables as your go-to food choice should you get hungry between meals. I recommend four servings of Everyday Vegetables per day in Phase 2, but, remember, it is fine to add an additional serving or two each day if you need a little extra food to chase away hunger.

Fruit: In Phase 2, we add two daily servings of fruit. I had suggested you avoid fruit in Phase 1 to reset your eating pattern, to help you to undo dietary damage done to your body in the past, and to start your body off with a clean slate prepared for the weight loss and resulting good health you so richly deserve. During Phase 1, I wanted you to avoid all sugar in order to help you break the control that sugar may have had on you and its inflammatory effect on your body. Now that you've done that for the first 15 days of Phase 1, you've strengthened your ability to avoid sweet foods, and you're ready to progress to a healthier, fuller way of eating, by adding fruit back into your diet. Eureka! How sweet it is!

Fruit is a nutrient-dense, high-volume food. What I mean by that is that fruit has a high concentration of nutrients and fiber, but it also contains lots of water. What's more, it's not calorically dense in the same way that fried chicken or a brownie is. With fruit (and to a greater extent, vegetables) you get filled up without taking in a lot of calories. Now, I never said fruit was calorie-free, so you do have to limit your intake of it. One of the first questions I ask clients who are not losing weight as quickly as they would like is how much fruit they are eating or fruit juice they are drinking. Often the answer is, "I eat as much as I like; it's good for you, right?" Yes, fruit is very good for you. But it also contains calories, so you can't eat unlimited amounts of it. Two servings a day strikes a good balance between nutrients and calories on a weight-loss diet, especially on the F-15 Plan.

As you add fruit to your daily menu, remember to choose a variety of different fruits. Rely mostly on whole fruits, such as apples, bananas, berries, cherries, citrus fruits, grapes, mango, melon, papaya, peaches, pears, pineapple, and plums. If you really enjoy dried fruit, have it very occasionally. The same goes for fruit juice, which contains lots of added sugar and little or no fiber. You're always better off having whole fruit.

You may be wondering whether to include bananas in your daily meal plan since they are sometimes mentioned as being high in sugar. It is true that bananas contain fruit sugar—more than some other fruits—and that eating them can raise blood sugar. However, because they contain fiber, their effect on blood sugar is much more modest than, say, candy or some other sugar-sweetened food. In addition, bananas pack a wallop of nutritional contributions in the form of potassium and magnesium. Both of these minerals are important for healthy muscles and help prevent muscle cramping during exercise. Potassium is also an important nutrient for people with hypertension, because it lowers blood pressure. However, because bananas are higher in calories than other fruits, limit them to a couple times a week or add half a banana to smoothies to save room for other lower-calorie fruits in your meal plan.

In case you're wondering, I recommend little or no fruit juice in the F-15 Plan. That's because commercially prepared fruit juice, with its added sugar, is a much poorer choice of nutrition than whole fruit. Fruit juices in general are not as healthy a food choice as the fruits they come from. Ounce for ounce, juices contain more calories and sugar and less fiber than whole fruits. And they don't stave off hunger; like other sugary beverages, your body barely notices them when you drink them, even though they are relatively high in calories. Compare a 6-ounce serving of apple juice to an apple with its skin. The apple juice provides 90 calories and a paltry 0.2 gram of fiber, while the apple contains 81 calories and 3.7 grams of fiber. Or a cup of orange juice is 112 calories compared to an orange at 60 calories. You see where I'm going, right? What's more, if you drink fruit juice when you're hungry, you'll still be hungry, but eat the apple or orange and you'll be pleasantly satiated.

Success Story

Morgan Murphree

72.6 pounds lost
29.6 inches lost overall

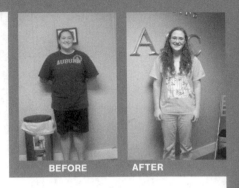

BEFORE **AFTER**

When I first met Morgan in my office, she was a high school student whose eating habits, like many of her peers, were terrible. When we first went over her food habits, her exact words were, "I eat anything and everything!"

What she lacked in fresh produce, she made up for with fast food and sweet tea (up to 40 ounces a day). On the rare occasion that she ate a salad, it was loaded with fatty ranch dressing. She ate very few vegetables and hardly any fruit.

Morgan was a beautiful, bright girl just waiting to break free from her shell, but the excess pounds that she carried on her tall frame stood in the way. Morgan thought herself unattractive, which couldn't have been further from the truth.

First I wanted to address the self-esteem issue that was such a heavy part of Morgan's self-concept. What my 28 years of experience as a nutritionist have taught me is this: I could prescribe all of the fruits and vegetables in the world, but if Morgan didn't see herself as worthwhile, it wouldn't make a difference.

I asked Morgan to find a picture of herself that she liked and to remember what it felt like to be that size. I asked her to place copies of the picture everywhere—on the mirror where she brushed her teeth, on her dresser, even on her smartphone.

We had to drastically change Morgan's diet, so she started following Phase 1 of the F-15 Plan. Once she had done one round of Phase 1, she began to see results. She was so gung ho that I suggested keeping up her newly found momentum by doing another 15-day round of Phase 1.

When we moved her to Phase 2 of the meal plan, she agreed to try fresh fruits for snacks. She realized that she had something of a sugar addiction, though, so we limited the fruit to one small fruit every other day. Since she loved ice cream, I taught her how to make a mock ice cream that I call Banana Nice Cream (page 192). Morgan loved it! I also provided Morgan with visuals to help her recognize foods by the correct portion sizes at home and away. Today as a college student, Morgan has moved from playing ball to doing CrossFit 5 days a week and is fully responsible for preparing and choosing her own foods. She handles it like a pro, even when she eats out with friends. I couldn't be more proud of her if she were my own daughter.

Morgan says, "Dr. Ro helped me to feel better about myself. Finally I'm not the largest person among my friends, and it feels great! The F-15 Plan gave me a new way to live. I'm so much happier with my life."

Low-fat dairy: Continue to include two servings per day of low-fat dairy. It contains various nutrients, including calcium, linked to supporting weight loss and keeping weight off after losing it, and two satiating ingredients: protein and fat, which help you feel fuller longer.

Fat: Keep up with the three servings of fat per day in Phase 2. Fat is a great hunger fighter, as long as you stay within the recommended intake. Make sure you're choosing the healthiest fats, such as cold-pressed extra virgin olive oil, peanut oil, and sesame oil, which are made without heat or chemical processing.

WATCH THESE PHASE 2 DIET TRAPS

In Phase 2, continue to avoid added sugar, grains, alcohol, and processed foods. Doing so will help you meet your weight-loss goals while boosting your health.

FIBER: YOUR SECRET SATIETY WEAPON

Vegetables and fruits are important parts of the F-15 Meal Plan. Not only do they contain amazing amounts of nutrients—vitamins, minerals, and antioxidants that boost health and reduce disease risks—but they are also excellent sources of dietary fiber. Nuts and seeds, as well as whole grains and legumes, also contribute significant amounts of fiber to your diet.

Dietary fiber is important because it adds bulk to your diet. This bulk helps you feel full, which is an extremely important benefit in a diet that is lower in calories than you're used to. Eating high-fiber foods makes food seem as if it has more calories. Eat 200 calories of a low-fiber food, and you'll feel hungrier sooner than you will if you eat 200 calories of a high-fiber food. Fiber is a great appetite suppressor because it fills you up more and keeps you feeling full longer, because of its bulk and the fact that it helps delay the absorption of food in your gastrointestinal system. And because it slows the absorption of food, fiber also gives the great benefit of stabilizing your blood sugar and insulin levels. Because it is bulky, fiber also helps to keep you regular. If you've ever been constipated, you know how wonderful regularity is!

Fiber has other benefits, as well. According to the American Institute for Cancer Research, eating a high-fiber diet may reduce the risk of certain diseases, such as heart disease, diabetes, and certain kinds of cancer, including cancers of the mouth, pharynx, larynx, esophagus, colon, rectum, and stomach. Fiber may even help to ward off lung disease; a 2016 study found better lung function in people who ate lots of fiber compared with those who didn't.

There are two types of dietary fiber: soluble and insoluble. **Soluble fiber** is found in certain whole grains (for example, barley and oats), legumes, fruits (such as apple skins), and vegetables. Soluble fiber is soft and sticky; when consumed, it dissolves and becomes gel-like once inside your body. As it goes through your digestive system, it binds to fatty substances (such as cholesterol) and moves them out of the body. Soluble fiber has a beneficial effect on blood sugar and insulin sensitivity, as well. **Insoluble fiber** is found in whole grains, dark leafy greens, seeds, nuts, legumes, fruits, and vegetables. Insoluble fiber passes through the intestines without being broken down, increasing the bulk of your stool and cleaning out your intestines along the way.

The current recommendation, according to the Institute of Medicine (IOM), is 25 grams of fiber per day for women and 38 grams per day for men. Don't worry about counting fiber grams in the F-15 Plan. If you eat the fruits, vegetables, legumes, nuts, seeds, and grains recommended in this plan, you'll get all the fiber you need.

One important thing to remember: If you are accustomed to eating a low-fiber diet, adding lots of fiber right away can result in gas, bloating, and cramping. If this happens to you, add fiber to your diet gradually. Make sure you drink plenty of water. Both soluble and insoluble fiber need water to do their jobs of slowing down the rate of filling up the stomach and preventing hunger (insoluble fiber) and of trapping and retaining water from the intestines to prevent constipation. Bottom line? Understand that fiber is a boon to your weight-loss process, and your body will adjust quickly to the added fiber, so any gas, bloating, or cramping will likely go away soon.

You may be wondering about fiber supplements; after all, if some is good, maybe more is better, right? Well, here's the deal. If you're closely following the F-15 Plan and getting all of the fruits, vegetables, nuts, seeds, legumes, and whole grains I recommend in each phase, you should be getting all of the fiber you need, and you shouldn't require additional fiber supplements. Foods are a much higher-quality source of fiber than fiber supplements because they contain not only fiber but also natural vitamins, minerals, antioxidants, and other important nutrients. However, if you have digestive health problems—such as irritable bowel disease, colitis, chronic diarrhea, or constipation—talk with your doctor about whether you could benefit from dietary fiber supplements.

FABULOUS PHYTOCHEMICALS

You've probably heard of phytochemicals, which are compounds in foods that help fight disease. But you may be wondering what exactly these compounds are and what they do. Here are a few things you should know about phytochemicals.

Phytochemical (or *plant chemical*) is an umbrella term that describes the numerous chemical compounds found in plant foods—fruits, vegetables, whole grains, legumes, seeds, and nuts. (*Phyto* means plant.) Common phytochemical names include antioxidants, flavonoids, carotenoids, phytonutrients, isoflavones, flavones, catechins, anthocyanins, polyphenols, isothiocyanates, and allyl sulfides.

Nutrition is an ever-evolving science. There are as many as 4,000 different kinds of phytochemicals in plant foods, and only a small number of them have been studied by nutrition researchers thus far. A variety of phytochemicals are found in various kinds—and colors—of plant foods. For example, red and purple vegetables and fruits are rich sources of anthocyanins, which have anti-inflammatory properties and have been found to reduce the risk of cardiovascular disease by boosting the condition of blood vessels. And the carotenoids found in orange and dark-green vegetables—such as carrots, sweet potatoes, spinach, and collard greens—help to strengthen vision, immunity, and the health of skin and bones.

Luckily, all you have to do is eat. Researchers know that many of the phytochemicals they've studied provide a range of health benefits, including a lower risk of diseases such as heart disease, diabetes, and some kinds of cancer. However, they aren't necessarily sure which phytochemicals do what. Luckily, we don't have to wait for scientists to study the effects of the 4,000 compounds. Instead, we can get all of their nutritional protection by eating a wide range of plant foods—like those recommended in the F-15 Plan. When it comes to fruits and vegetables, you can't go wrong following the recommendation to eat from the rainbow, choosing produce that's red, yellow, orange, dark green, and purple. Keep this in mind when you make salads of fruits or vegetables: The more colors you include, the better!

The Phase 2 **F-15** Meal Plan

As we've discussed, this second phase of the F-15 Plan includes four servings of protein, four servings of vegetables, two servings of fruit, two servings of low-fat dairy, and three servings of fat per day. Although I recommend having protein and vegetables at each meal and snack, the way you choose to allocate your daily servings is up to you. As in Phase 1, you can choose to design your own daily menus or use my 15-Day Meal Plans. Go with whatever works best for you!

PHASE 2, WEEK I

Notes about the Meal Plans

- Meal plans include approximately 1,200 to 1,400 calories per day.
- Foods listed in **bold** have recipes in the recipe section.
- Asterisks (*) denote there is a variation in the ingredient and/or its amount for that recipe for that specific meal and day.
- Have lemon water with each meal and snack. Lemon water is made with water and the juice of two lemon wedges. Mint lemon water is made by adding 2 tablespoons chopped fresh mint. Basil lemon water is made by adding 2 tablespoons chopped fresh basil. Cucumber lemon water is made by adding 3 to 5 slices cucumber. Or you can mix any combination of these herbs with lemon and/or cucumber for a refreshing drink.

Day 1

MEAL OR SNACK	FOODS	F-15 SERVINGS
Breakfast	1 serving **Melon and Prosciutto Breakfast Salad** (page 167) 1 cup green tea 16 ounces lemon water	1½ Proteins 1 Vegetable 1 Fruit 1 Fat
Morning Snack	1 serving **Ice Cream Smoothie** (page 168) 20 ounces lemon water	½ Protein 1 Fruit 1 Dairy
Lunch	Tossed Salad with Tuna (3 ounces drained canned water-packed tuna over tossed salad made with ¼ cup shredded red cabbage, ¼ cup grated carrots, 1 cup mixed greens, 5 cherry tomatoes, and 2 tablespoons fat-free Italian dressing) 20 ounces lemon water	1 Protein 1 Vegetable
Afternoon Snack	Stuffed Celery with Herbed Cottage Cheese (2 stalks celery stuffed with ½ cup 1% cottage cheese mixed with 2 tablespoons chopped basil) 20 ounces lemon water	1 Dairy
Dinner	1 serving **Black Bean Pasta with Shrimp in Red Curry Sauce** (page 186) Tossed Salad (2 cups mixed greens tossed with 1 serving **Dr. Ro's Salad Dressing,** page 181) 20 ounces lemon water	1 Protein 2 Vegetables 2 Fats
Evening Snack	20 ounces lemon water	
	Total for the Day	4 Proteins 4 Vegetables 2 Fruits 2 Dairy 3 Fats

Day 2

MEAL OR SNACK	FOODS	F-15 SERVINGS
Breakfast	1 serving **Power Breakfast Parfait** (page 172) 2 ounces extra-lean Canadian bacon, broiled with 1 spray olive oil cooking spray 1 cup green tea 16 ounces lemon water	1 Protein 1 Fruit 1 Dairy
Morning Snack	Nuts and Berries 12 almonds ½ cup halved strawberries 20 ounces lemon water	1 Fruit 1 Fat
Lunch	Kale Patty Wrap with Sriracha Mayo (Cut 1 Dr. Praeger's Kale Veggie Burger in half and top each burger half with 3 hard-cooked egg whites and 1 tablespoon reduced-fat olive oil mayonnaise mixed with ¼ teaspoon Sriracha chili sauce, divided; wrap each half of burger with toppings in 1 leaf of lettuce) 20 ounces lemon water	1 Protein 1 Vegetable 1 Fat
Afternoon Snack	1 serving **Smoked Trout and Cottage Cheese Sliders** (page 114) 20 ounces lemon water	1 Protein 1 Vegetable 1 Dairy
Dinner	1 serving **Chicken with Tomatoes and Olives** (page 116) Tossed Salad (2 cups mixed greens tossed with 2 tablespoons fat-free Italian dressing) 1 sweet potato, baked (or microwaved for 7 to 8 minutes), with a sprinkle of ground cinnamon 20 ounces lemon water	1 Protein 2 Vegetables 1 Fat
Evening Snack	20 ounces lemon water	
	Total for the Day	4 Proteins 4 Vegetables 2 Fruits 2 Dairy 3 Fats

Day 3

MEAL OR SNACK	FOODS	F-15 SERVINGS
Breakfast	Veggie-Kale Egg White Omelet	2 Proteins
	(3 egg whites, ¼ cup sliced mushrooms, ¾ cup chopped kale, 1 tablespoon chopped red onion, and ¼ cup cherry tomatoes, halved, cooked in 1 tablespoon extra virgin olive oil)	1 Vegetable
		1 Dairy
	2 ounces extra-lean Canadian bacon, broiled with 1 spray olive oil cooking spray	1 Fat
	1 cup nonfat milk	
	1 cup green tea	
	16 ounces lemon water	
Morning Snack	20 ounces lemon water	
Lunch	Tossed Salad with Turkey Breast	1 Protein
	(4 ounces roast turkey breast over tossed salad made with 1 cup mixed greens; ¼ cup cucumber slices; 5 cherry tomatoes, halved; and 1 tablespoon white balsamic vinegar mixed with ½ tablespoon extra virgin olive oil)	1 Vegetable
		1 Fat
	20 ounces lemon water	
Afternoon Snack	Minted Fresh Fruit	1 Fruit
	(½ cup strawberries, halved, with a sprig of fresh mint, chopped)	
	20 ounces lemon water	
Dinner	1 serving **Sesame Salmon with Apple Slaw** (page 188)	1 Protein
	12 spears asparagus, steamed	2 Vegetables
	Spinach Salad (1 cup fresh spinach, ¼ tablespoon walnuts, 1 ounce crumbled feta cheese, and ¼ cup sliced Granny Smith apples tossed with ¼ tablespoon extra virgin olive oil mixed with 1 tablespoon white balsamic vinegar)	1 Fruit
		1 Dairy
		1 Fat
	20 ounces lemon water	
Evening Snack	20 ounces lemon water	
	Total for the Day	4 Proteins
		4 Vegetables
		2 Fruits
		2 Dairy
		3 Fats

Day 4

MEAL OR SNACK	FOODS	F-15 SERVINGS
Breakfast	1 serving **Savory Tomato Breakfast Bowl** (page 173) 2 ounces extra-lean Canadian bacon, broiled with 1 spray olive oil cooking spray 1 cup green tea 16 ounces lemon water	1 Protein 1 Vegetable 1 Dairy 1 Fat
Morning Snack	20 ounces lemon water	
Lunch	1 serving **Turkey and Herbed Cottage Cheese Tomato Wrap** (page 178) 1 small apple 20 ounces lemon water	1 Protein 1 Vegetable 1 Fruit 1 Dairy 1 Fat
Afternoon Snack	½ cup strawberries, halved 20 ounces lemon water	1 Fruit
Dinner	Grilled Chicken Breast (6 ounces boneless, skinless chicken breast grilled with ½ tablespoon extra virgin olive oil) 1 serving **Sautéed Spinach** (page 189) Tossed Salad (2 cups mixed greens tossed with 2 tablespoons fat-free Italian dressing) 20 ounces lemon water	2 Proteins 2 Vegetables 1 Fat
Evening Snack	20 ounces lemon water	
	Total for the Day	4 Proteins 4 Vegetables 2 Fruits 2 Dairy 3 Fats

Day 5

MEAL OR SNACK	FOODS	F-15 SERVINGS
Breakfast	1 serving **Yummy Omelet Squares** (page 175)	1 Protein
	1 slice extra-lean Canadian bacon, broiled with 1 spray olive oil cooking spray	1 Vegetable
	1 cup green tea	
	16 ounces lemon water	
Morning Snack	1 serving **Red Grapefruit–Jalapeño Water Infusion** (page 177)	½ Fruit
		1 Dairy
	1 piece part-skim mozzarella string cheese	
	20 ounces lemon water	
Lunch	1 serving **Warm Steak Salad** (page 183)	1 Protein
	½ cup blueberries	1 Vegetable
	20 ounces lemon water	1 Fruit
		1 Fat
Afternoon Snack	1 piece part-skim mozzarella string cheese	1 Protein
	3 hard-cooked egg whites	1 Dairy
	20 ounces lemon water	
Dinner	Vegetable-Shrimp Stir-Fry	1 Protein
	(¼ cup bamboo shoots, 1 egg white, ½ cup sliced mushrooms, ½ cup nonstarchy mixed vegetables, 4 ounces peeled and deveined shrimp, and 2 teaspoons reduced-sodium soy sauce stir-fried in 1 tablespoon toasted sesame oil)	2 Vegetables
		2 Fat
	Tossed Salad (1 cup mixed greens tossed with 1 tablespoon extra virgin olive oil mixed with 2 tablespoons white balsamic vinegar)	
	20 ounces lemon water	
Evening Snack	¼ red grapefruit	½ Fruit
	20 ounces lemon water	
	Total for the Day	4 Proteins
		4 Vegetables
		2 Fruits
		2 Dairy
		3 Fats

Day 6

MEAL OR SNACK	FOODS	F-15 SERVINGS
Breakfast	1 serving **Pick-Me-Up Green Smoothie** (page 171) 1 hard-cooked egg white 1 cup green tea 16 ounces lemon water	1 Protein 1 Vegetable 1 Fruit
Morning Snack	1 serving **Smoked Trout and Cottage Cheese Sliders** (page 114) (use ½ a cucumber) 20 ounces lemon water	1 Protein ½ Vegetable 1 Dairy
Lunch	1 serving **Lunchtime Turkey Rolls** (page 112) (add 2 teaspoons extra virgin olive oil) 1 orange 20 ounces lemon water	1 Protein 1 Vegetable 1 Fruit 1 Dairy 1 Fat
Afternoon Snack	20 ounces lemon water	
Dinner	Baked Lemon-Dill Salmon (4 ounces salmon baked using 1 tablespoon extra virgin olive oil, ¼ cup chopped fresh dill, ¼ tablespoon garlic powder, ¼ teaspoon ground black pepper, a dash of salt, and juice of ½ lemon) ½ cup chopped broccoli florets, steamed ½ serving **15-Minute Spaghetti Squash** (page 115) 20 ounces lemon water	1 Protein 1½ Vegetables 2 Fats
Evening Snack	20 ounces lemon water	
	Total for the Day	4 Proteins 4 Vegetables 2 Fruits 2 Dairy 3 Fats

Day 7

MEAL OR SNACK	FOODS	F-15 SERVINGS
Breakfast	1 serving **Tropical Protein Smoothie** (page 170)	½ Protein
	1 cup green tea	1 Fruit
	16 ounces lemon water	1 Dairy
Morning Snack	Turkey Lettuce Wraps	½ Protein
	(2 ounces roast turkey breast and 1 teaspoon mustard mixed with 1 tablespoon reduced-fat olive oil mayonnaise divided and wrapped in 2 leaves lettuce)	1 Fat
	20 ounces lemon water	
Lunch	1 serving **Black Bean Spaghetti with Tomatoes and Basil** (page 184)	1 Protein
		2 Vegetables
	Tossed Salad (2 cups mixed greens tossed with 2 tablespoons fat-free Italian dressing)	1 Fat
	20 ounces lemon water	
Afternoon Snack	2 hard-cooked egg whites	1 Protein
	1 piece part-skim mozzarella string cheese	1 Dairy
	20 ounces lemon water	
Dinner	1 serving **Asian-Style Beef with Asparagus** (page 185)	1 Protein
	½ sweet potato, microwaved, topped with ⅛ teaspoon ground cinnamon	2 Vegetables
	20 ounces lemon water	1 Fat
Evening Snack	1 small apple (optional)	1 Fruit
	20 ounces lemon water	
	1 cup chamomile tea	
	Total for the Day	4 Proteins
		4 Vegetables
		2 Fruits
		2 Dairy
		3 Fats

PHASE 2, WEEK 2

Day 1

MEAL OR SNACK	FOODS	F-15 SERVINGS
Breakfast	1 serving **Fat-Burner Smoothie** (page 169)	1½ Proteins
	1 hard-cooked egg	½ Vegetable
	1 cup green tea	1½ Fruits
	16 ounces lemon water	1 Dairy
Morning Snack	20 ounces lemon water	
Lunch	1 serving **Quick-n-Easy Tuna Lunch** (page 179)	1½ Proteins
	Tossed Salad (1 cup mixed greens tossed with 1 serving **Dr. Ro's Salad Dressing,** page 181)	1½ Vegetables
		1 Fat
	20 ounces lemon water	
Afternoon Snack	½ cup 1% cottage cheese	¼ Fruit
	¼ kiwifruit	1 Dairy
	20 ounces lemon water	
Dinner	1 serving **Grape Chicken*** (page 182) (use ¼ cup grapes)	1 Protein
		2 Vegetables
	1 serving **Sautéed Spinach** (page 189) (made with 1 tablespoon extra virgin olive oil and 1 teaspoon trans fat–free buttery spread)	¼ Fruit
		2 Fats
	1 sweet potato, baked (or microwaved for 7 to 8 minutes), topped with 2 teaspoons trans fat–free buttery spread and sprinkled with ¼ teaspoon ground cinnamon	
	20 ounces lemon water	
Evening Snack	20 ounces lemon water	
Total for the Day		4 Proteins
		4 Vegetables
		2 Fruits
		2 Dairy
		3 Fats

Day 2

MEAL OR SNACK	FOODS	F-15 SERVINGS
Breakfast	Yogurt with Berries, Nuts, and Cinnamon (1 container [5.3 ounces] nonfat plain Greek yogurt topped with 1 ounce [2 tablespoons] chopped walnuts, ¼ teaspoon ground cinnamon, and ½ cup sliced strawberries) 1 hard-cooked egg 1 cup green tea 16 ounces lemon water	1 Protein 1 Fruit 1 Dairy 1 Fat
Morning Snack	Basil hummus (4 tablespoons hummus mixed with 2 tablespoons chopped basil) 1 cup cucumber slices 20 ounces lemon water	1 Protein 1 Vegetable
Lunch	1 serving **Lunchtime Turkey Rolls** (page 112) (add 1 teaspoon extra virgin olive oil) Tossed Salad (1 cup mixed greens and ½ cup cherry tomatoes, halved, tossed with 2 tablespoons fat-free Italian dressing) 20 ounces lemon water	1 Protein 1 Vegetable 1 Dairy 1 Fat
Afternoon Snack	20 ounces mint-cucumber lemon water	
Dinner	1 serving **Sesame Salmon with Apple Slaw** (page 188) (add 1 teaspoon extra virgin olive oil) 12 spears asparagus, steamed 1 peach 20 ounces lemon water	1 Protein 2 Vegetables 1 Fruit 1 Fat
Evening Snack	20 ounces basil lemon water	
	Total for the Day	4 Proteins 4 Vegetables 2 Fruits 2 Dairy 3 Fats

Day 3

MEAL OR SNACK	FOODS	F-15 SERVINGS
Breakfast	1 serving **Smoky Salmon Breakfast Scramble** (page 176) ½ cup blueberries 1 cup green tea 16 ounces lemon water	1½ Proteins 1 Vegetable 1 Fruit 1 Fat
Morning Snack	1 cup grapes 1 piece part-skim mozzarella string cheese 20 ounces lemon water	1 Fruit 1 Dairy
Lunch	Grilled Chicken Salad (3 ounces boneless, skinless chicken breast, grilled, served over a salad made with 2 cups mixed greens; ¼ cup cucumber slices; 5 cherry tomatoes, halved; and 2 tablespoons fat-free Italian dressing) 20 ounces lemon water	1 Protein 1 Vegetable
Afternoon Snack	Yogurt with Cinnamon and Nuts (1 container [5.3 ounces] nonfat plain Greek yogurt topped with 1 ounce chopped walnuts and ¼ teaspoon ground cinnamon) 20 ounces lemon water	1 Dairy 1 Fat
Dinner	Broiled Lemon-Dill Fish (6 ounces orange roughy, broiled or grilled, with 5 sprigs fresh dill, chopped; juice of 3 lemon wedges; and salt and ground black pepper to taste and drizzled with ½ tablespoon extra virgin olive oil) 1 serving **Broccoli, Tomato, and Onion Sauté** (page 190) 1 serving **Garlic-Ginger Sautéed Bok Choy** (page 191) 20 ounces lemon water	1½ Proteins 2 Vegetables 1 Fat
Evening Snack	20 ounces lemon water	
	Total for the Day	4 Proteins 4 Vegetables 2 Fruits 2 Dairy 3 Fats

Day 4

MEAL OR SNACK	FOODS	F-15 SERVINGS
Breakfast	1 serving **Tuscan Breakfast Salad with Canadian Bacon** (page 108) 1 cup green tea 16 ounces lemon water	2 Proteins 1½ Vegetables 1 Fat
Morning Snack	1 ounce low-fat cheddar or Colby cheese ¾ cup strawberries, halved 20 ounces lemon water	1½ Fruits 1 Dairy
Lunch	1 serving **Turkey and Herbed Cottage Cheese Tomato Wrap** (page 178) 1 cup 1% milk 20 ounces lemon water	1 Protein 1 Vegetable 1 Dairy 1 Fat
Afternoon Snack	20 ounces basil-cucumber lemon water	
Dinner	1 serving **Grape Chicken** (page 182) served over ½ cup cooked spaghetti squash Tossed Salad (2 cups mixed greens tossed with 1 serving **Dr. Ro's Salad Dressing,** page 181) 20 ounces of mint lemon water	1 Protein 1½ Vegetables ½ Fruit 1 Fat
Evening Snack	20 ounces mint-cucumber lemon water	
	Total for the Day	4 Proteins 4 Vegetables 2 Fruits 2 Dairy 3 Fats

Day 5

MEAL OR SNACK	FOODS	F-15 SERVINGS
Breakfast	1 serving **Power Breakfast Parfait** (page 172)	1 Protein
	3 hard-cooked egg whites	1½ Fruits
	1 cup green tea	1 Dairy
	16 ounces lemon water	
Morning Snack	Turkey Lettuce Wraps	1 Protein
	(3 ounces roast turkey breast and 2 teaspoons mustard divided and wrapped in 3 leaves lettuce)	1 Vegetable
	20 ounces lemon water	
Lunch	Turkey Cheeseburger Lettuce Wraps with Chili Mustard	1 Protein
		1 Vegetable
	(3-ounce ground turkey patty [93% lean], broiled with 1 tablespoon extra virgin olive oil, ½ tablespoon Worchestershire sauce, ½ tablespoon teriyaki sauce, and ¼ teaspoon each salt, pepper, and garlic powder and topped with 1 slice [1 ounce] low-fat Colby or cheddar cheese, ½ tablespoon mustard mixed with ½ teaspoon Sriracha chili sauce, and 2 tomato slices, divided and wrapped in 2 leaves butterhead lettuce)	1 Dairy
	20 ounces lemon water	
Afternoon Snack	20 ounces basil-cucumber lemon water	
Dinner	1 serving **Citrus-Ginger Halibut** (page 187)	1 Protein
	12 spears asparagus, steamed	2 Vegetables
	Tossed Salad (2 cups mixed greens, ½ cup cucumber slices, and ½ cup cherry tomatoes tossed with 2 tablespoons fat-free Italian dressing)	½ Fruit
		2 Fats (*Note:* Halibut has 16 g of fat without added fat during cooking, hence the "2 Fats.")
Evening Snack	20 ounces lemon water	
	Total for the Day	4 Proteins
		4 Vegetables
		2 Fruits
		2 Dairy
		3 Fats

Day 6

MEAL OR SNACK	FOODS	F-15 SERVINGS
Breakfast	Prosciutto Breakfast Salad with Egg Whites (2 cups mixed greens, 2 slices prosciutto di Parma, ¼ cup sliced avocado, sections from ½ red grapefruit, and 3 hard-cooked egg whites dressed with 1 tablespoon toasted sesame oil and 1 tablespoon white balsamic vinegar) 1 cup green tea 20 ounces lemon water	2 Proteins 1 Vegetable 1 Fruit 1 Fat
Morning Snack	Herbed Cottage Cheese (½ cup 1% cottage cheese mixed with 1 tablespoon chopped fresh basil) 20 ounces lemon water	1 Dairy
Lunch	Tossed Salad with Tuna (3 ounces drained canned water-packed tuna over tossed salad made with 1 cup shredded red cabbage; ¼ cup grated carrots; 10 cherry tomatoes, halved; and 2 tablespoons fat-free Italian dressing) 20 ounces lemon water	1 Protein 1 Vegetable
Afternoon Snack	1 container (4 ounces) nonfat plain yogurt 1 cup sliced strawberries 20 ounces mint lemon water	1 Fruit 1 Dairy
Dinner	Baked Lemon-Garlic Chicken (4 ounces boneless, skinless chicken breast baked with juice of ¼ lemon; 1 tablespoon extra virgin olive oil; 3 cloves garlic, minced; and ⅛ teaspoon each salt and ground black pepper) 12 spears asparagus, sautéed in 1 tablespoon extra virgin olive oil Tossed Salad (2 cups mixed greens and ½ cup cherry tomatoes tossed with 2 tablespoons fat-free Italian dressing) 20 ounces lemon water	1 Protein 2 Vegetables 2 Fats
Evening Snack	20 ounces mint lemon water	
	Total for the Day	4 Proteins 4 Vegetables 2 Fruits 2 Dairy 3 Fats

Day 7

MEAL OR SNACK	FOODS	F-15 SERVINGS
Breakfast	1 serving **Spicy Spinach-Lentil Breakfast Bowl** (page 174) ½ cup 1% cottage cheese ½ cup halved strawberries 1 cup green tea 20 ounces lemon water	1½ Proteins 1 Vegetable 1 Fruit 1 Dairy 1 Fat
Morning Snack	½ cup 1% cottage cheese 1 peach	1 Fruit 1 Dairy
Lunch	Spicy Salmon Lettuce Wraps (1 tablespoon whipped low-fat cream cheese mixed with ¼ teaspoon Sriracha chili sauce, 4 ounces grilled salmon, ¼ cup sliced avocado, and ½ cup spinach divided and wrapped in 5 leaves lettuce) 20 ounces basil lemon water	1 Protein 1 Vegetable 1 Fat
Afternoon Snack	20 ounces basil lemon water	
Dinner	1 serving **15-Minute Fish with Cucumber Sauce** (page 113) (made with 5 ounces fish) 1 cup chopped bok choy, steamed 1 serving **Sautéed Spinach** (page 189) 20 ounces lemon water	1½ Proteins 2 Vegetables 1 Fat
Evening Snack	20 ounces cucumber lemon water	
	Total for the Day	4 Proteins 4 Vegetables 2 Fruits 2 Dairy 3 Fats

Day 8

MEAL OR SNACK	FOODS	F-15 SERVINGS
Breakfast	Yogurt with Cinnamon and Nuts (1 container [5.3 ounces] nonfat Greek yogurt mixed with 1 teaspoon vanilla extract and topped with 1 ounce chopped walnuts and ¼ teaspoon ground cinnamon) 1 hard-cooked egg 1 cup green tea 20 ounces lemon water	1 Protein 1 Dairy 1 Fat
Morning Snack	½ serving **Pick-Me-Up Green Smoothie** (page 171) 2 hard-cooked egg whites 20 ounces basil lemon water	1 Protein 1 Vegetable 1 Fruit
Lunch	Broiled Salmon Spinach Salad with Mandarin Orange Dressing (3 ounces salmon, broiled, over salad made with 2 cups fresh spinach, 1 ounce goat cheese, ½ table-spoon chopped walnuts, and 1 serving **Mandarin Orange Vinaigrette**, page 180) ½ cup tangerine sections 20 ounces lemon water	1 Protein 1 Vegetable 1 Fruit 1 Dairy 1 Fat
Afternoon Snack	20 ounces basil lemon water	
Dinner	Grilled Chicken with Black Bean Spaghetti (2 ounces chicken breast, grilled, with 2 ounces black bean spaghetti, cooked according to package direc-tions, topped with sauce made from 1 clove garlic, minced; 2 teaspoons extra virgin olive oil; ½ cup chopped tomatoes; and 1 tablespoon chopped fresh basil and sprinkled with 1 tablespoon grated Parmesan cheese) ½ cup chopped broccoli florets, steamed 20 ounces lemon water	1 Protein 2 Vegetables 1 Fat
Evening Snack	20 ounces mint lemon water	
	Total for the Day	4 Proteins 4 Vegetables 2 Fruits 2 Dairy 3 Fats

Grocery List, Phase 2

PANTRY ITEMS AND STAPLES

See list in Phase 1 (page 103)

PHASE 2, WEEK I

MEATS AND FISH

Bacon (Hormel Black Label maple bacon): 1 slice

Beef flank steak: ½ pound

Boneless, skinless chicken breast: ½ pound

Canadian bacon, extra lean: ¼ pound

Lean turkey salami: 4 ounces

Prosciutto di Parma: 1 package

Roast turkey breast (sliced): ¾ pound

Salmon: ½ pound

Shrimp: ½ pound

Trout: ¼ pound

VEGGIE BURGERS

Dr. Praeger's Kale Veggie Burgers: 1 box

DAIRY

Almond milk (unsweetened): ½ cup

Cottage cheese (1%): 3 cups

Feta cheese: 1½ ounces

Greek yogurt (organic, nonfat, plain): 1 container (5.3 ounces)

Provolone cheese (reduced fat): 1 slice (1 ounce)

Parmesan cheese (reduced fat): ¼ pound (check your pantry list before putting this item in your basket)

String cheese (part-skim mozzarella): 4 (small package)

Yogurt (organic, low fat, plain): 3 containers (4 ounces each)

FRUITS AND VEGETABLES

Apples: 2

Asparagus: 2 pounds

Avocado: ¾ cup

Bananas: 3

Bell peppers: 2

Blueberries: ½ cup

Broccoli: ½ cup

Brussels sprouts: 1 cup

Butterhead lettuce: 1 head

Cabbage (savoy): 1 small head

Carrots: 2

Celery: 1 head

Chives: 1

Cucumbers: 4

Flat-leaf parsley: 1 bunch

Fresh ginger: 1 piece

Garlic cloves: 5

Grapefruit (red): 1

Green beans: ¾ cup or 1 frozen package (10 ounces)

Green leaf lettuce: 1 head

Jalapeño pepper: 1

Kale: 1¾ cups

Kiwifruit: 1

Lemons: 10

Mango: 1 large

Mixed greens: 1½ cups

Mixed vegetables: ½ cup

Mushrooms: ½ cup

Orange: 1

Peaches (frozen): ½ cup

Pineapple: 2 slices

Pomegranate seeds: ½ cup

Portobello mushrooms: ½ cup

Red cabbage: ¼ cup

Red onion: 1 large

Romaine lettuce: 2 cups

Scallions: 2

Spaghetti squash: 1

Spinach (fresh): 4½ cups

Spinach (frozen): 1 package (10 ounces)

Strawberries: 1 pint

Sweet potatoes: 2 small

Tangerines: 2

Tomatoes (cherry): 3 cups

Tomatoes (Italian or plum): 4

Watermelon: 1 cup

Zucchini: 1

PHASE 2, WEEK 2

MEATS AND FISH

Boneless, skinless chicken breasts: 1 pound

Canadian bacon, extra lean: 2 ounces

Ground turkey (93% lean): ¼ pound

Haddock: ¼ pound

Halibut: ¼ pound

Lean turkey salami: 4 ounces

Orange roughy: ½ pound

Prosciutto di Parma: 2 slices

Roast turkey breast (sliced): ⅓ pound

Salmon: ¾ pound

Salmon lox: 2 ounces

DAIRY

Almond milk (unsweetened): 1 pint or quart

Cottage cheese (1%): 4 cups

Cheddar or Colby cheese (low fat): 2 ounces

Cream cheese (whipped, low fat): 2 tablespoons

Goat cheese: 1 ounce

Greek yogurt (organic, nonfat, plain): 3 containers (5.3 ounces each)

Provolone cheese (reduced fat): 1 slice (1 ounce)

Sargento reduced-fat Italian blend shredded cheese: ¼ cup

String cheese (part-skim mozzarella): 1 piece

Yogurt (organic, low fat, plain): 4 containers (4 ounces each)

FRUITS AND VEGETABLES

Apple: 1

Asparagus: 1 pound

Avocado: 1

Bananas: 2

Bell peppers: 1

Blueberries: ½ cup

Bok choy: 2 cups

Broccoli: 1½ cups

Brussels sprouts: ½ cup

Butterhead lettuce: 1 head

Carrots: 1

Chives: 1

Cucumber slices: 3 cups

Fresh ginger: 1 piece

Garlic cloves: 9

Grapefruit: ½

Grapes: 2 cups

Green leaf lettuce: 1 head

Kale: 4½ cups

Kiwifruit: 3

Lemons: 10

Lettuce: 1 head

Mixed greens: 6 cups

Mushrooms: ¼ cup

Orange: 1

Peaches: 2

Pineapple: 1 cup plus 1 slice

Portobello mushrooms: ½ cup

Red cabbage: 1 cup

Red onion: 1 large

Savoy cabbage: 2 cups

Scallions: 1

Spinach (fresh): 7 cups

Spinach (frozen): 1 package
(10 ounces)

Strawberries: 4 cups

Tangerines: 4

Tomatoes (cherry): 2½ cups

Tomatoes (Italian or plum): 2

The Phase 2 Recipes

To help you stay on track with this second phase of the F-15 Plan, I've created recipes for delicious, filling foods that fit perfectly into this phase. A few of my personal favorites are the Black Bean Pasta with Shrimp in Red Curry Sauce (page 186), the Melon and Prosciutto Breakfast Salad (page 167), and the Sesame Salmon with Apple Slaw (page 188). The quick and easy breakfast bowls, most made in 15 minutes, are to live for! I could go on, but it would be so much better for you to dig in and get started making them for yourself. I can't wait for you to put them to them to test!

MELON AND PROSCIUTTO BREAKFAST SALAD WITH FRIED EGG

SERVES 1

2 cups mixed greens

2 tablespoons roughly chopped fresh basil

1 tablespoon toasted sesame oil

2 tablespoons white balsamic vinegar

1 cup diced watermelon

1 slice prosciutto di Parma

1 fried egg

In a salad bowl, add the mixed greens, basil, oil, and vinegar and toss well. Top with the watermelon, prosciutto, and egg.

F-15 SERVINGS:	
1½	Proteins
1	Vegetable
1	Fruit
1	Fat

NUTRITION INFORMATION:	
Calories:	359
Fat:	24 g
Carbs:	29 g
Protein:	13 g

ICE CREAM SMOOTHIE

SERVES 1

½ banana, frozen

½ cup chopped mango

¼ scoop hemp protein concentrate

1 teaspoon vanilla extract

1 teaspoon almond extract

1 cup 1% milk

3 or 4 ice cubes

Dash of ground cinnamon

In a blender, combine the banana, mango, hemp protein, vanilla, almond extract, milk, and ice cubes. Blend until the desired consistency. Add water as needed for smoothness. Top with the cinnamon.

F-15 SERVINGS:

1	Protein
1	Fruit
1	Dairy

NUTRITION INFORMATION:

Calories:	265
Fat:	4 g
Carbs:	40 g
Protein:	16 g

FAT-BURNER SMOOTHIE

SERVES 1

5 thin slices fresh ginger
  (1" in diameter)

⅓ scoop hemp protein concentrate

1 small kiwifruit

Juice of ½ lemon

½ cup frozen or fresh pineapple
  chunks

1 cup fresh spinach

1 container (4 ounces) low-fat plain
  yogurt

4 ice cubes

In a blender, combine the ginger, hemp protein, kiwi, lemon juice, pineapple, spinach, yogurt, and ice cubes. Blend until the desired consistency. Add water as needed for smoothness.

F-15 SERVINGS:

1	Protein
1	Vegetable
2	Fruits
1	Dairy

NUTRITION INFORMATION:

Calories:	203
Fat:	4 g
Carbs:	30 g
Protein:	15 g

TROPICAL PROTEIN SMOOTHIE

SERVES 1

¼ teaspoon almond extract

½ banana, frozen

½ cup frozen unsweetened sliced peaches

½ scoop hemp protein concentrate

½ cup 1% milk

½ container (2 ounces) low-fat plain yogurt

3–4 ice cubes

⅛ teaspoon ground cinnamon

In a blender, combine the almond extract, banana, peaches, hemp protein, milk, yogurt, and ice cubes. Blend until smooth. Top with the cinnamon.

F-15 SERVINGS:

½	Protein
1	Fruit
1	Dairy

NUTRITION INFORMATION:

Calories:	303
Fat:	6 g
Carbs:	43 g
Protein:	23 g

PICK-ME-UP GREEN SMOOTHIE

SERVES 1

½ scoop Amazing Grass Organic Wheat Grass Powder

½ scoop hemp protein concentrate

5 slices fresh ginger

1 cup roughly chopped kale

1 cup fresh spinach

½ kiwifruit

2 slices fresh pineapple

Juice of ¼ lemon

1 cup water

3 ice cubes

¼ teaspoon matcha green tea powder (optional, for energy boost)

In a blender, combine the wheatgrass powder, hemp protein, ginger, kale, spinach, kiwi, pineapple, lemon juice, water, and ice cubes. Blend on high until smooth. For extra punch and an energy boost, add the green tea powder after pouring the blended smoothie into a tall glass. Stir vigorously until fully blended.

F-15 SERVINGS:

½	Protein
2	Vegetables
1	Fruit

NUTRITION INFORMATION:

Calories:	220
Fat:	3 g
Carbs:	37 g
Protein:	14 g

POWER BREAKFAST PARFAIT

SERVES 1

1 container (5.3 ounces) nonfat plain Greek yogurt

¼ teaspoon matcha green tea powder

½ cup strawberries, sliced

½ banana, sliced

1 tablespoon ground flaxseed

Sprig of fresh mint for garnish (optional)

1. In a small bowl, combine the yogurt and green tea powder.

2. In a clear glass or plastic glass or bowl, layer the yogurt, strawberries, banana, and half of the flaxseed.

3. Top with the remaining flaxseed and the mint, if desired.

F-15 SERVINGS:

1	Fruit
1	Dairy

NUTRITION INFORMATION:

Calories:	252
Fat:	6 g
Carbs:	27 g
Protein:	21 g

SAVORY TOMATO BREAKFAST BOWL

SERVES 1

1 cup fresh spinach

2 tablespoons Classico Sun-Dried Tomato Pesto

½ cup cherry tomatoes, halved

1 container (4 ounces) low-fat plain yogurt

Dash of salt (optional)

¼ avocado, cut into chunks

2 tablespoons chopped fresh basil

½ tablespoon roasted, unsalted pumpkins seeds

1. In a medium nonstick skillet coated with cooking spray over medium heat, cook the spinach for 4 minutes, or until tender.

2. In a medium bowl, combine the spinach, pesto, tomatoes, and yogurt. Add the salt, if desired.

3. Top with the avocado, basil, and pumpkin seeds.

F-15 SERVINGS:

1	Vegetable
1	Dairy
1	Fat

NUTRITION INFORMATION:

Calories:	284
Fat:	14 g
Carbs:	27 g
Protein:	16 g

SPICY SPINACH-LENTIL
BREAKFAST BOWL

SERVES 1

3 egg whites

1 tablespoon toasted sesame oil, divided

2 cups frozen spinach, thawed and water squeezed out

¼ teaspoon ground cumin

½ teaspoon ground coriander

¼ cup cooked lentils

½ tablespoon red wine vinegar

2 teaspoons reduced-sodium soy sauce

Toasted sesame seeds (optional)

1. In a nonstick skillet coated with cooking spray over medium-high heat, scramble the egg whites for a few minutes, or until soft and formed but not hard scrambled. Remove and set aside.

2. In the same skillet, add ½ tablespoon of the oil, the spinach, cumin, and coriander and cook, stirring frequently, for 5 minutes, or until the spinach is tender.

3. Stir the lentils and reserved scrambled egg whites into the spinach mixture to heat through.

4. In a medium bowl, whisk together the vinegar, soy sauce, and the remaining ½ tablespoon oil and toss the lentil and spinach mixture in the sauce.

5. Sprinkle with toasted sesame seeds, if desired, and serve.

F-15 SERVINGS:	
1½	Proteins
1	Vegetable
1	Fat

NUTRITION INFORMATION:	
Calories:	259
Fat:	15 g
Carbs:	13 g
Protein:	19 g

YUMMY OMELET SQUARES

SERVES 4

6 eggs, separated into yolks and whites

½ teaspoon onion powder

¼ teaspoon salt

¼ teaspoon ground black pepper

¼ teaspoon garlic powder

4 cups canned stewed tomatoes

½ zucchini, cut into quarters lengthwise and then sliced

1. Preheat the oven to 350°F. Coat an 8" x 8" x 2" baking dish with nonstick cooking spray.

2. In a medium bowl, beat the egg yolks, onion powder, salt, pepper, and garlic powder for 4 minutes, or until thick and lemon colored. Set aside.

3. In a separate bowl, beat the egg whites until soft peaks form. Fold into the egg yolks.

4. Spread the egg mixture evenly into the baking dish. Bake for 22 minutes, or until a knife inserted near the center comes out clean.

5. Meanwhile, in a saucepan over medium heat, bring the tomatoes and zucchini to a boil. Reduce the heat to low, cover, and simmer for 5 minutes, or until the zucchini is tender.

6. To serve, cut the omelet into quarters and top with the sauce.

F-15 SERVINGS:

1	Protein
1	Vegetable

NUTRITION INFORMATION (PER SERVING):

Calories:	177
Fat:	7 g
Carbs:	18 g
Protein:	12 g

SMOKY SALMON BREAKFAST SCRAMBLE

SERVES 1

1 tablespoon extra virgin olive oil

1 cup chopped kale

½ cup chopped portobello mushrooms

¼ cup sliced red onion

1 egg white

1 egg

2 tablespoons chopped fresh basil

½ teaspoon chopped fresh thyme

¼ teaspoon ground black pepper

1 ounce smoked salmon (lox), chopped into bite-size pieces

1. In a nonstick skillet over medium-high heat, warm the oil. Cook the kale, mushrooms, and onion until tender.

2. In a medium bowl, whisk together the egg white and egg. Pour into the veggie mixture and add the basil, thyme, and pepper. Scramble until the eggs are scrambled to desired doneness. Add the lox.

F-15 SERVINGS:

1½	Protein
1	Vegetable
1	Fat

NUTRITION INFORMATION:

Calories:	354
Fat:	25 g
Carbs:	11 g
Protein:	25 g

RED GRAPEFRUIT–JALAPEÑO WATER INFUSION

SERVES 2

¼ red grapefruit, sliced

¼ cup chopped fresh basil

¼ jalapeño pepper, seeded and sliced (wear plastic gloves when handling)

20 ounces water

In a pitcher, combine the grapefruit, basil, jalapeño, and water. Cover and infuse overnight.

F-15 SERVINGS:

½	Fruit

NUTRITION INFORMATION (PER SERVING):

Calories:	14
Carbs:	3 g

15 MINUTE RECIPE

TURKEY AND HERBED COTTAGE CHEESE TOMATO WRAPS

SERVES 1

6 leaves butterhead lettuce

3 ounces roast turkey breast, torn into small pieces

2 teaspoons spicy brown mustard

⅛ teaspoon garlic powder

½ cup 1% cottage cheese

2 tablespoons chopped fresh basil

1 tablespoon chopped chives

1 cup fresh baby spinach

6 thin slices tomato

¼ cup sliced avocado

3 lemon wedges

1. Lay out the lettuce leaves.

2. In a medium bowl, combine the turkey, mustard, garlic powder, cottage cheese, basil, and chives until well mixed.

3. Divide and layer the spinach and tomato onto the lettuce leaves. Divide and spread on the turkey mixture. Top with the avocado slices and a squeeze of lemon juice. Roll up and secure with toothpicks.

Note: If making ahead of time, pack the filling separately in an airtight container and wrap lettuce leaves in damp paper towels and store in a plastic bag.

F-15 SERVING:	
1	Protein
1	Vegetable
1	Dairy
1	Fat

NUTRITION INFORMATION:	
Calories:	306
Fat:	8 g
Carbs:	10 g
Protein:	42 g

QUICK-N-EASY TUNA LUNCH

SERVES 1

3 ounces drained canned
  water-packed tuna

1 cup cherry tomatoes

½ teaspoon smoked paprika

½ cup drained canned black beans

¼ teaspoon salt (optional)

¼ teaspoon ground black pepper
  (optional)

2 tablespoons chopped fresh basil

1. In a nonstick skillet over medium-high heat, cook the tuna, tomatoes, and smoked paprika, stirring occasionally, for 5 minutes, or until the tomatoes break down and become saucy.

2. Add the beans and cook until heated through. Season with the salt and pepper, if desired. Toss in the basil.

F-15 SERVING:

1½	Proteins
1	Vegetable

NUTRITION INFORMATION:

Calories:	239
Fat:	4 g
Carbs:	27 g
Protein:	30 g

MANDARIN ORANGE VINAIGRETTE

SERVES 1

½ tablespoon extra virgin olive oil

2 tablespoons white balsamic vinegar

¼ cup tangerine sections

In a small bowl, whisk together the oil and vinegar. Add the tangerines (also called mandarin oranges) and crush with a fork to desired consistency. Drizzle over spinach or salad greens of your choice.

Note: This recipe can be used for any fruity vinaigrette you desire, such as mango, raspberry, blueberry, peach, or watermelon.

F-15 SERVINGS:	
¼	Fruit
¾	Fat

NUTRITION INFORMATION:	
Calories:	106
Fat:	7 g
Carbs:	17 g

DR. RO'S SALAD DRESSING

SERVES 1

1½ tablespoons white balsamic vinegar

1 tablespoon extra virgin olive oil

In a small bowl, whisk together the vinegar and oil.

F-15 SERVINGS:	
1	Fat

NUTRITION INFORMATION:	
Calories:	135
Fat:	14 g
Carbs:	8 g

GRAPE CHICKEN

SERVES 1

---

3 ounces boneless, skinless chicken breast

1 cup fat-free, low-sodium chicken broth

1 teaspoon cornstarch

¼ teaspoon dried or chopped fresh mint

¼ cup seedless red or green grapes, halved

1. In a large nonstick skillet coated with cooking spray over medium heat, cook the chicken for 8 to 10 minutes, turning to brown evenly, or until the chicken is no longer pink. Remove from the skillet and keep warm.

2. In a small bowl, combine the broth, cornstarch, and mint. Add to the skillet and cook, stirring frequently, until thickened and bubbly. Cook and stir for 2 minutes. Stir in the grapes and cook for 2 minutes, or until heated through. To serve, pour the sauce over the chicken.

F-15 SERVINGS:

1	Protein
½	Fruit

NUTRITION INFORMATION:

Calories:	139
Fat:	2 g
Carbs:	10 g
Protein:	20 g

WARM STEAK SALAD

SERVES 1

¼ cup green beans

3 cloves garlic, finely chopped, divided

3 ounces beef flank steak, trimmed of all fat

¼ teaspoon salt

¼ teaspoon ground black pepper

1 tablespoon extra virgin olive oil

2 tablespoons white balsamic vinegar

1 teaspoon Dijon mustard

¼ cup cucumber slices

1 cup shredded romaine lettuce

¼ cup cherry tomatoes, halved

3 teaspoons chopped fresh thyme

¼ cup chopped fresh flat-leaf parsley

1. In a shallow microwaveable bowl or dish, place the green beans with 2 tablespoons of water. Cover the dish tightly with plastic wrap and make a 1" slit on the top of the wrap to allow steam to escape. Microwave on high for 3 to 4 minutes, or until the green beans are bright green and firm but tender.

2. Rub three-quarters of the garlic into the steak on both sides. In a nonstick skillet coated with cooking spray over medium-high heat, cook the steak for 4 minutes on each side, or until preferred degree of doneness. Remove from the skillet, let stand for 5 minutes, and then cut across the grain into thin slices. Sprinkle with the salt and pepper.

3. In a small bowl, combine the oil, vinegar, mustard, and the remaining one-quarter of the garlic and whisk to a smooth consistency.

4. In a large bowl, add the cucumber, lettuce, tomatoes, thyme, and parsley. Toss with half the dressing. Arrange in a shallow salad or dessert bowl or plate. Add the green beans and steak slices. Drizzle the remaining dressing over the salad.

F-15 SERVINGS:	
1	Protein
1	Vegetable
1½	Fats

NUTRITION INFORMATION:	
Calories:	347
Fat:	20 g
Carbs:	25 g
Protein:	27 g

BLACK BEAN SPAGHETTI WITH TOMATOES AND BASIL

SERVES 1

2 ounces black bean spaghetti

1 tablespoon extra virgin olive oil

1 cup cherry tomatoes, halved

¼ cup chopped fresh basil

1 clove garlic, minced

1 tablespoon grated Parmesan cheese

1. Cook the spaghetti according to package instructions. Drain and return to the saucepan.

2. In the saucepan, toss the cooked pasta with the oil, tomatoes, basil, and garlic.

3. Top with the cheese and serve.

F-15 SERVINGS:	
1	Protein
1	Vegetable
1	Fat

NUTRITION INFORMATION:	
Calories:	350
Fat:	18 g
Carbs:	6 g
Protein:	28 g

ASIAN-STYLE BEEF WITH ASPARAGUS

SERVES 1

4 tablespoons reduced-sodium teriyaki marinade

¼ cup fat-free, low-sodium beef broth

¼ teaspoon Thai chili garlic paste

1 tablespoon toasted sesame oil

½ cup diagonally cut asparagus pieces (1" long)

½ cup diagonally cut green bean pieces (1" long)

4 cloves garlic, minced

4 ounces beef flank steak, trimmed of all fat and cut into bite-size pieces

¼ cup cherry tomatoes, halved

¼ cup chopped scallions

1. In a small bowl, combine the teriyaki marinade, broth, and chili garlic paste. Set aside.

2. In a skillet over high heat, warm the oil. Cook the asparagus, green beans, and garlic for 3 minutes, or until the asparagus and green beans are crisp-tender.

3. Push the vegetables to the side of the skillet. Add the steak and cook, stirring frequently, for 2 minutes, or until done.

4. Add the reserved marinade, tomatoes, and scallions. Reduce the heat to low and simmer for 1 minute. Serve.

F-15 SERVINGS:

1	Protein
1½	Vegetables
1	Fat

NUTRITION INFORMATION:

Calories:	409
Fat:	22 g
Carbs:	11 g
Protein:	28 g

BLACK BEAN PASTA
WITH SHRIMP IN
RED CURRY SAUCE

SERVES 1

2 ounces black bean spaghetti

2 ounces shrimp, peeled and deveined

¼ cup chopped yellow bell pepper

¼ cup chopped red bell pepper

½ tablespoon extra virgin olive oil

⅛ cup low-fat unsweetened coconut milk

1 teaspoon grated fresh ginger

¼ teaspoon salt

¼ teaspoon ground black pepper

¼ tablespoon Thai-brand red curry paste

½ teaspoon ground coriander

1 tablespoon grated reduced-fat Parmesan cheese

1. Cook the spaghetti according to package instructions. Drain.

2. Meanwhile, in a medium skillet over medium heat, cook the shrimp and bell peppers in the oil for 4 to 5 minutes, or until the shrimp are pink.

3. In a saucepan over medium heat, bring the coconut milk, ginger, salt, black pepper, curry paste, and coriander to a boil for about 5 minutes, or until thickened. Remove from the heat.

4. Add the pasta and mix well. Add the shrimp and bell peppers. Top with the cheese and serve.

F-15 SERVINGS:

1	Protein
½	Fat

NUTRITION INFORMATION:

Calories:	383
Fat:	15 g
Carbs:	28 g
Protein:	35 g

CITRUS-GINGER HALIBUT

SERVES 1

Grated peel of ½ lemon

Grated peel of ½ orange

Juice of ½ orange

Juice of 1 lemon

½ tablespoon extra virgin olive oil

1 tablespoon chopped fresh mint

½ teaspoon grated fresh ginger

¼ teaspoon salt

¼ teaspoon ground black pepper

4 ounces halibut

¼ teaspoon paprika

Slice of lemon for garnish

Sprig of flat-leaf parsley for garnish

1. Preheat the oven to 400°F. Coat a baking dish with cooking spray.

2. In a medium bowl, combine the lemon peel, orange peel, orange juice, lemon juice, oil, mint, ginger, salt, and pepper.

3. Add the fish to the marinade and toss to coat. Marinate for 15 to 20 minutes.

4. Place the fish in the baking dish, drizzle with the marinade, and sprinkle with the paprika.

5. Cover and bake for 10 to 15 minutes, or until the fish flakes with a fork.

6. Garnish with the lemon slice and parsley.

F-15 SERVINGS:	
1	Protein
½	Fruit
1	Fat

NUTRITION INFORMATION:	
Calories:	304
Fat:	23 g
Carbs:	11 g
Protein:	17 g

SESAME SALMON
WITH APPLE SLAW

SERVES 1

3 ounces salmon

¼ teaspoon salt, plus more to taste

¼ teaspoon ground black pepper, plus more to taste

⅓ tablespoon extra virgin olive oil

2 cups shredded savoy cabbage

½ cup thinly sliced Brussels sprouts

¼ cup shredded carrots

¼ Gala apple, cut into bite-size pieces

1 small scallion, thinly sliced

2 ounces nonfat plain Greek yogurt

1 tablespoon lemon juice

¼ ounce toasted sesame seeds

Sprig of fresh flat-leaf parsley

Lemon slice

1. Season the salmon with the ¼ teaspoon salt and the ¼ teaspoon pepper. In a large nonstick skillet over medium-high heat, warm the oil. Cook the salmon 3 to 4 minutes per side, or until the fish becomes opaque and flakes with a fork.

2. Meanwhile, in a medium bowl, toss together the cabbage, Brussels sprouts, carrots, apple, scallion, yogurt, lemon juice, and more salt and pepper to taste.

3. Gently sprinkle the sesame seeds over the salmon and serve with the slaw. Garnish with the parsley and lemon slice.

F-15 SERVINGS:

1	Protein
1½	Vegetables
¼	Fruit
¼	Dairy
⅓	Fat

NUTRITION INFORMATION:

Calories:	363
Fat:	20 g
Carbs:	21 g
Protein	26 g

SAUTÉED SPINACH

SERVES 2

2 cups fresh or 1 package
(10 ounces) frozen and thawed
spinach

½ tablespoon extra virgin olive oil

3 cloves garlic, thinly sliced

¼ teaspoon salt

¼ teaspoon ground black pepper

1 lemon wedge

1. If using frozen spinach, squeeze out the water.

2. In a nonstick skillet over medium-high heat, warm the oil. Cook the garlic for about 2 minutes.

3. Cook the spinach for 4 minutes, or until tender.

4. Sprinkle with the salt and pepper and serve with the lemon wedge.

F-15 SERVINGS:

1	Vegetable
½	Fat

**NUTRITION INFORMATION
(PER SERVING):**

Calories:	80
Fat:	7 g
Carbs:	4 g
Protein:	2 g

BROCCOLI, TOMATO, AND ONION SAUTÉ

SERVES 1

¼ tablespoon extra virgin olive oil

½ cup chopped broccoli

2 tablespoons sliced red onion

1 tomato, diced

2 tablespoons Sargento reduced-fat Italian blend shredded cheese

1. In a large skillet over medium heat, warm the oil for 2 to 3 minutes. Add the broccoli and onion and cook for 7 to 8 minutes, or until tender.

2. Add the tomatoes and cook, stirring frequently, for 2 to 3 minutes, or until the tomatoes are hot.

3. Top with the cheese and serve.

F-15 SERVINGS:

1	Vegetable
¼	Fat

NUTRITION INFORMATION:

Calories:	66
Fat:	4 g
Carbs:	6 g
Protein:	3 g

GARLIC-GINGER SAUTÉED BOK CHOY

SERVES 1

½ tablespoon sesame oil

2 cloves garlic, finely chopped

2 cups bite-size bok choy pieces

½ teaspoon finely chopped fresh ginger

1 tablespoon reduced-sodium soy sauce

1. In a large nonstick skillet or wok over medium heat, warm the oil for 2 to 3 minutes. Cook the garlic for 1 to 2 minutes, or until fragrant.

2. Add the bok choy, ginger, and soy sauce and cook for 5 to 7 minutes, or until the bok choy leaves become bright green and the stalks are slightly translucent.

F-15 SERVINGS:	
1	Vegetable
½	Fat

NUTRITION INFORMATION:	
Calories:	44
Fat:	3 g
Carbs:	1 g
Protein:	2 g

BANANA NICE CREAM

SERVES 1

½ banana, frozen (see note)

2 tablespoons unsweetened almond milk

¼ teaspoon ground cinnamon

½ teaspoon sunflower seeds or crunchy almond butter or peanut butter (optional)

In a small food processor, add the frozen banana and almond milk. Pulse to the desired consistency. Sprinkle with the cinnamon and the sunflower seeds or nut butter, if desired.

Note: Keep frozen bananas on hand for this recipe and other smoothies.

F-15 SERVINGS:	
1	Fruit

NUTRITION INFORMATION:	
Calories:	57
Fat:	0.5 g
Carbs:	14 g
Protein:	1 g

Your 15-Minute Moves for Phase 2

In Phase 1, you tried some of my favorite 15-Minute Moves. Now that you're building up your fitness level, it's time to move on to some slightly more challenging moves. Exercise directions follow the workouts.

SUMO SQUATS

LOWER BODY (GLUTEAL AND QUADRICEPS MUSCLES)

Step 1: Place your feet in a wide stance with your toes turned out at an even angle.

Step 2: With your legs in a wide stance and your hips over the center of your feet, start to lower your body by pushing your hips back as if to sit in a chair, bending your knees and pushing your body weight into your heels. Remember to keep your chest up and shoulders back while bending from your hips, and *always* keep a neutral spine for protection.

Step 3: Sit as low as possible (the goal is to have your legs parallel with the floor, but go as low as is comfortable for you, and *never* exceed your comfort level). As you sit, raise your arms in front of your body or raise them over your head to assist with balance.

Step 4: Pause at the bottom of the motion before driving through your heels to stand. Keep your knees behind your toes and your weight in your heels to prevent injury.

PUSHUPS

UPPER BODY (TRICEPS, SHOULDERS)

Step 1: Start by lying face down with your hands on the floor shoulder-width apart, palms down. Keep your weight distributed between your hands and feet, with your toes pointed toward the floor. Prop your body up to a plank position, keeping rigid and straight.

Step 2: Lower your body until your chest nears the floor at the bottom of the movement, and return to the start position (bend your knees and push up from the knee if you need help lifting your entire body). Remember to move in a smooth, fluid motion using and tightening your core. At the top of the pushup, exhale as you lower your body back to the floor, and inhale as you lift off for the next rep. Be proud of yourself! You're doing what you thought you couldn't do. Prove to

---

Tabata Workout #2

TOTAL TIME: 15 MINUTES

1. Sumo Squats and Pushups—20 seconds of Sumo Squats and 10 seconds of rest; 20 seconds of Pushups and 10 seconds of rest; repeat the sequence for 4 minutes.

REST FOR 1 MINUTE.

2. Alternating Lunges (page 128) and Alternating V-Ups— 20 seconds of Alternating Lunges and 10 seconds of rest; 20 seconds of Alternating V-Ups and 10 seconds of rest; repeat the sequence for 4 minutes.

REST FOR 1 MINUTE.

3. Jumping Jacks and Plank Jacks—20 seconds of Jumping Jacks and 10 seconds of rest; 20 seconds of Plank Jacks and 10 seconds of rest; repeat the sequence for 4 minutes.

STRETCH. YOU'RE DONE!

CONGRATS! YOU MADE IT! YOU'RE AWESOME!

---

yourself every day that you can do something more. You're stronger than you think!

Congrats! You just did one repetition!

BEGINNER LEVEL: Keep your knees bent to push up from your knees.

HIIT Workout #2

TOTAL TIME: 15 MINUTES

1. 1 minute of Jumping Jacks (beginner: 30 seconds)

2. 30 seconds of Plank Jacks (beginner: 15 seconds)

3. Rest for 30 seconds

4. 1 minute of Alternating (forward) Lunges (page 128) (beginner: 30 seconds)

5. 30 seconds of Pushups (page 194) (beginner: 15 seconds)

6. Rest for 30 seconds

7. 1 minute of Alternating V-Ups (beginner: 30 seconds)

8. 30 seconds of Sumo Squats (page 193)

9. Rest for 30 seconds

10. 1 minute of Jumping Jacks

11. 30 seconds of Plank (page 124)

12. Rest for 30 seconds

13. Repeat the cycle until you've reached the 15-minute mark. Go!

STRETCH. YOU'RE DONE!

CONGRATS! YOU MADE IT! YOU'RE AWESOME!

ALTERNATING V-UPS

ABS (CORE STRENGTH), UPPER BODY

Step 1: Lie on your back with your arms extended above your head, palms facing the ceiling, legs extended in front of your body, and toes pointed toward the ceiling. Raise your upper body, bringing both arms up off the floor to touch the toes of one foot at a time, beginning with the left foot.

Step 2: Return to the start position, then raise your upper body to touch the toes of your right foot. Squeeze your abdominal muscles as you reach for your toes. Exhale as you return to the start position.

ADVANCED LEVEL: From the start position, raise both arms to touch both legs at once. Add a weight to each hand for the advanced level.

JUMPING JACKS

CARDIO

Step 1: Standing with your feet together and your arms by your sides, jump, raising your arms above your head and bringing your palms together at the top of the movement. Then return your feet to the floor with a smooth coordinated motion.

Step 2: Return to the starting position, bringing your arms back to your side, and repeat the motion until you have completed the number of jumping jacks needed to progress to your next exercise.

BEGINNER LEVEL: Step one leg at a time out to the side while reaching your arms above your head.

PLANK JACKS

CORE, GLUTEAL MUSCLES (GLUTES FOR BACKS OF THIGHS)

Step 1: Start in a pushup position with your feet together, toes pointed toward the floor.

Step 2: Do a quick jump while in a pushup position, extending your legs outward as far as you can and landing softly on your toes. (Beginners: If you're not ready to jump yet, using one leg at at a time, touch your toes outward, and then return to the start position.)

Step 3: Jump again, bringing your feet back together and repeat.

AMRAP Workout #2

TOTAL TIME: 15 MINUTES

1. Jab-Cross Squat Combo—Do 15 reps.

2. Pushups (page 194)—Do 15 reps.

3. Crunches (page 127)—Do 15 reps.

4. Plank Jacks—Do 15 reps.

5. Rest as needed between rounds. Repeat cycle, doing as many rounds as possible for 15 minutes.

STRETCH. YOU'RE DONE!

CONGRATS! YOU MADE IT! YOU'RE AWESOME!

Kickboxing Move

JAB-CROSS SQUAT COMBO

UPPER BODY, LOWER BODY, CARDIO

Step 1: Stand with your feet firmly planted on the ground. Place your right foot in front of your left foot and your left foot slightly behind.

Step 2: Keeping your elbows at your sides and your hands in front of your face, punch with your right arm and then pull back to the start.

Step 3: Squat. On the rise from squatting, returning to the start position, add an Alternating Side Kick with your right foot.

Step 4: Follow through with a punch with your left arm, and then pull back to the start.

Step 5: Squat. On the rise from squatting, returning to the start position, add an alternating side kick with your left foot.

Success Story

Joyce Wilson

40 pounds lost
18.9 inches lost overall

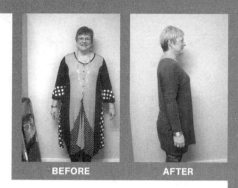

BEFORE   **AFTER**

When Joyce came to my office, she said she "needed a professional" to help her set and reach her weight-loss goals. She was going to the gym every day, but her eating habits had kept her from "accomplishing anything" from all of her hard work.

Joyce co-owned a small business with her husband of 35 years, and then, suddenly, her best friend and business partner fell ill and died after just 7 short months, leaving her to run the business alone. Joyce had already been working long hours, but caring for her husband those 7 months took its toll. Then, as if that wasn't enough stress and pressure, her ailing elderly mother, whom she still cares for, needed a caretaker, too.

When Joyce told me about all the challenges in her life, I completely understood. I wondered, how much can one person be expected to take? Hell, I wanted to offer her a dinner made of doughnuts and chocolate cake! But I knew she had come to me for help and with the hope that somehow I could get her set on a sound diet and meal plan that would at least take off her extra physical weight. I knew that I could provide what she wanted, but her emotional challenges needed to be addressed if the diet was to work.

Because Joyce was grieving and still reeling from the loss of her husband and caring for her mother, we had to allow her time and give her the tools she needed to process her feelings. We worked on ways to identify Joyce's specific feelings and put them in perspective.

Joyce's time was limited because, like so many other women, she wore so many hats. She needed to be able to prepare meals in short periods of time, so we worked on developing 15-minute meals, grab-n-go meals and snacks, and food prep routines for the few minutes of downtime she could steal on weekends.

Finally, the junk food had to go. Her meal plan, like yours, began with no added sugar, grains, fried foods, soda, or even fruit for the first 15 days. She balked at first since this was the way she was used to eating but conceded that since she didn't have the answers, she might as well try my way. I jokingly reminded her that "when at first you don't succeed, do what your coach told you to do in the first place." Around my office, we have an expression (which my uncle used to use on me): "If I tell you the moon is green cheese, you run and get crackers!"

Joyce now says, "I have gained all the self-worth and confidence I need to face the challenges of my new life. Losing weight was hard enough, but Dr. Ro's support got me through a really tough time."

In the Next Chapter:
Phase 3 of the **F-15** Plan

You're making amazing progress! You've completed Phase 1 of the F-15 Plan, and by now you've already done Phase 2. Yaaaay for you! Next on deck is the final phase of the F-15 Plan: Phase 3, Coast and Maintain. During the 15-day Phase 3 plan, you'll continue to burn fat and lose weight while having even more food choices. And I've got even more amazing recipes, 15-Minute Moves, 15-Minute Stress Busters, and lots of other great tools for you. I'm so proud of you for making it this far. Let's keep going, and you'll move even closer to meeting your goals!

Chapter 6

PHASE 3: COAST AND MAINTAIN

You had everything you needed to succeed
in this life when you were created.
Take a look inside. It's still there.
—Dr. Ro

Woo-hoo! You've made your way through Phase 1 and Phase 2 of the F-15 Plan. Now it's time to advance to Phase 3. Your results should be looking pretty impressive. Your metabolism is in high gear, and your body is busy burning fat every day. As far as your weight goes, you are likely seeing some notable changes on the scale and around your waist, hips, thighs, and wherever else you carry extra fat. By this point, many people who follow the F-15 Plan report weight loss of about 10 to 12 pounds, give or take a few. The higher your weight when you started the F-15 Plan, the more likely you are to drop pounds quickly. If your weight is coming off a bit more slowly than that, don't give up. All bodies are different, and some want very much to hold on to excess weight.

If you're not losing as quickly as you had hoped, I encourage you to cycle back to repeat Phase 1 and to stay on that phase for 15 to 30 days if necessary. Then after seeing the results that you want, cycle up to Phase 2 again. Phase 3 is the meal plan that incorporates all of the foods that will support weight maintenance. It's a plan that you can sustain for life. That's why I call it Coast and Maintain, because you will use this plan to coast through the rest of your life while maintaining your weight loss. But as long as you are in weight-loss mode, your best bets are Phases 1 and 2, in that order. I would also advise that you reread my guidelines in Phases 1 and 2 and make sure that you're following them closely. Reconsider whether or not you are sticking to the recommended number of servings and correct portions. Answer these questions as you contemplate your next step. Are you choosing the right serving sizes? Are you staying away from junk food, sugary snacks, and alcoholic beverages?

Soon you can expect to reach your first 15-pound weight-loss goal, if you haven't reached it already. Many people have by this time. Kudos to you if you have! If you set out to lose just 15 pounds, you will be reaching your goal. If you want to lose more than 15 pounds, cycle back and forth between Phases 1 and 2 until you lose as much weight as you desire. If you start to gain a few extra pounds, if you become stuck in a plateau, or if you want to give your metabolism a kick in the pants, you can always go back to Phase 1 and Phase 2 to stoke your metabolic fires. Use Phase 3 for your final maintenance.

In Phase 2, we continued focusing on fat burning, but we also shifted the focus a little to allow you to adapt to your new diet, and we added more delicious food choices to your daily meal plan. We continue that in Phase 3. In this cycle of the diet, you get to enjoy even more variety. And you will continue to eat a well-balanced diet with controlled portion sizes of health-giving foods—which is the heart and soul of the F-15 Plan. During Phase 3, you'll expand your choices even further by adding in whole grain foods several days per week.

Exercise will remain an important component of your life during Phase 3, as well. You will continue to work exercise into your daily life by using my 15-Minute Moves. You can keep using the moves from Phase 1 and Phase 2, and you can try some new Phase 3 moves, too.

And, of course, Phase 3 provides the menu-planning help you need, with a 15-Day Meal Plan and 15 fabulous F-15 recipes that all fit like a glove into the Phase 3 guidelines.

The Phase 3 Servings Plan

Phase 3 includes many of the same great choices found in Phases 1 and 2. For example, you'll continue to eat plenty of power-packed foods in each meal, including lean protein, nutrient-rich vegetables, fruit, low-fat dairy, and fats. But during this phase, you'll get even more food with the inclusion of whole grains. To help you capitalize on the energy-sustaining power of the combination of lean protein mixed with whole grains, I've included whole grains in your daily meal plan 3 days a week.

Success Story

Jason Thomason

25.2 pounds lost
5.5 inches lost overall

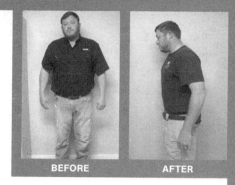

BEFORE   **AFTER**

Jason is a thirty-something firefighter who also owns a landscaping business. Jason had been fairly active, but around the age of 30 his metabolism started slowing down and he became sluggish. Jason said he noticed a slight bulge in his midsection. He came to me feeling worn down and unhappy with the way his body looked. He said that having gained a few extra pounds had slowed him down physically, and he wasn't pleased with that result.

We started by cutting out the empty calories—sodas and beer—Jason had been drinking daily. We replaced them with 100 ounces of lemon water a day to reduce inflammation. His knees were weak, and reducing inflammation in the body can help with inflammatory-based health problems.

We added more monounsaturated fatty acids (MUFAs) to his diet to reduce his growing belly. MUFAs are helpful for people who store fat in the belly area because they help you to feel satiated. They also reduce inflammation. They are far healthier than highly processed, sugar-laden foods, and studies show they can increase insulin sensitivity and help to stabilize blood sugar.

Jason followed Phase 1 of the F-15 Plan for 30 days (two rounds of 15 days each), a choice anyone on the plan can make to help enhance results or overcome a plateau. Jason needed to give his weight loss an extra boost to prove to himself that he could do it. He started to see a difference in his weight after the first 15 days, but to keep it going at that rate, he agreed to continue with Phase 1 for 15 more days, and it paid off. During his first month, he lost 15 pounds. He still had 10 to 15 pounds left to lose, according to his goal weight.

Next we progressed to a hybrid version of Phase 2, adding a serving of high-fiber complex carbs every other day for 30 days. He lost 25.2 pounds and 5.5 inches overall, with most of the inches lost in the belly area. Jason and I were both astonished by his progress. "My weight can affect my job as a firefighter and my business. I value them both too much to compromise. Dr. Ro's F-15 Plan really helped me to get back in shape. I don't feel tired all the time like I used to."

It's this simple: Each day during Phase 3, you'll eat a total of 15 servings of food: four servings of protein (lean meat, poultry, fish, beans, nuts, seeds, and eggs), three or four servings of vegetables (depending on whether you eat grains that day), two servings of fruit, two servings of low-fat dairy foods, three servings of fat, and one serving of whole grains 3 days a week on "grain days." That comes to a total of 15 servings per day.

PHASE 3 SERVINGS

During Phase 3 of the F-15 Plan, 3 days a week will be "grain days." On these days, you will replace one serving of vegetables with one serving of whole grains.

Here are the foods you will eat.

ON GRAIN DAYS:

- ✓ 4 servings of protein
- ✓ 3 servings of vegetables
- ✓ 2 servings of fruit
- ✓ 2 servings of low-fat dairy
- ✓ 3 servings of fat
- ✓ 1 serving of whole grains

TOTAL: **15 servings per day**

ON NONGRAIN DAYS:

- ✓ 4 servings of protein
- ✓ 4 servings of vegetables
- ✓ 2 servings of fruit
- ✓ 2 servings of low-fat dairy
- ✓ 3 servings of fat

TOTAL: **15 servings per day**

(For a full review of serving sizes, see the tables in Chapter 3.)

BEHIND THE SERVINGS

As in Phases 1 and 2, the Phase 3 eating plan has been carefully designed to be as effective and as easy to follow as possible. Here's a quick guide to what you'll be eating in Phase 3.

Protein: Once again, protein is the centerpiece of your daily meal plan. The protein found in meat, poultry, fish, eggs, nuts, legumes, and seeds helps keep your metabolism revved up, supports your body as it loses fat and builds muscle, lines you up for optimal weight loss, and helps keep hunger at bay.

Vegetables: As in the previous two phases of the F-15 Plan, vegetables will continue to be an important part of your day's menus. Vegetables, which are high in fiber and water, help fill you up and keep you satiated. They should be in most or all of your meals and snacks. During Phase 3, you'll continue to enjoy Everyday Vegetables and Occasional Vegetables. As in Phase 2, feel free to have two servings per week of Occasional Vegetables, and continue to count them in your F-15 daily serving tally. For a reminder of which vegetables are which, see the lists on pages 56 to 57.

Fruit: In Phase 3, you'll continue to include two daily servings of fruit. Not only is fruit naturally sweet and delicious, but it's a nutrient-dense, high-volume food that contains lots of water. Fruit fills you up without lots of calories. As you plan your daily meals, remember to choose a variety of different whole fruits of different colors.

Low-fat dairy: As in previous phases, Phase 3 continues to include two servings per day of low-fat dairy, which contains various nutrients to boost your weight loss, such as calcium and two very satisfying components: protein and fat, both of which help you feel fuller longer.

Fat: Continue having three servings of fat per day in Phase 3. Fat helps keep you from getting hungry. Stick with the healthiest fats, such as cold-pressed olive oil, peanut oil, sesame oil, which are made without heat or chemical processing.

Whole grains: In Phase 3, you can have three weekly servings of whole grains. On the days in which you have a serving of whole grains, skip one of your vegetable servings. Once you're well established eating a healthy diet—which by now, as you progress to Phase 3, you've accomplished—you can incorporate all of the foods that comprise the well-balanced diet that you will enjoy for the rest of your life. A completely balanced diet for most healthy people should include whole grains for energy, to stabilize blood sugar, and for satiety—all important factors to achieve your weight-loss goals.

I had suggested that you avoid whole grains in the past two phases because even though they provide vitamins, minerals, and fiber to your diet, they are also high in calories and carbohydrates. At this stage of the process, your only job, as it relates to choosing whole grains, is to be selective about the ones you include in your diet.

You want to choose whole grains that contribute the greatest amount of nutrients and fiber, with the least amount of calories. You want them to be whole, unprocessed, and sprouted when possible. That is the trick to including whole grains in your weight-loss meal plan. And to give yourself the biggest benefit of stabilized blood sugar, the more fiber the better.

Remember to choose the most nutritious of grains. One of the best is sprouted grain bread. As I mentioned, my favorite choice (for reasons outlined in Chapter 3) is Ezekiel 4:9 sprouted 100% whole grain bread.

Some diet plans cut out whole grains entirely. But current research does not support this inclination. For example, a 2015 study published in the journal *JAMA Internal Medicine* found that eating whole grains appears to reduce the risk of cardiovascular disease and early death. Harvard researchers analyzed the eating patterns of nearly 75,000 women in the Nurses' Health Study and 44,000 men in the Health Professionals Follow-Up Study and found that every 1-ounce serving of whole grains was associated with 5 percent lower rates of early death and 9 percent lower rates of death from cardiovascular disease. Other studies have found additional benefits to eating whole grains. The trick is not to eat too many of them and to choose whole grains that are packed with nutrients. Some great whole grains to try include red quinoa; barley; whole grain couscous; rolled or steel-cut oats; wild rice; and brown, black, or red rice. And if you like pasta, choose low-carb, high-protein options such as kelp, soba, or buckwheat noodles and shirataki noodles. (For more on grain choices, see Chapter 3.)

Here are serving sizes for whole grains.

- Breads (sliced bread, bagels, biscuits, cornbread, English muffins, tortillas, etc.): 1 slice or a 1-ounce portion

Success Story

Sherri Shepherd

40 pounds lost

6.5 inches in the midsection lost

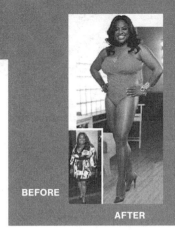

BEFORE

AFTER

Sherri is a busy mom with an even busier schedule and career. She is a bicoastal actress/comedian who requires lots of energy to work in TV and film. Sherri does not really cook, and eating the right foods for her high-octane schedule and managing her constantly fluctuating weight posed a challenge. And to add to her already full plate, she has diabetes. Sherri wanted to lose weight in a healthy way that would help keep her blood sugar stable.

First we had to keep Sherri from eating at soul food joints, her second home. She loved plates of fried chicken, collard greens, mac and cheese, candied yams, and corn bread. Obviously, that wouldn't do. Soul food, cooked the right way, can fit into a healthy diet, but we needed to rearrange and resize her plate. We replaced those soul-food favorites with some healthier choices, such as sautéed collards without meat, baked chicken rather than fried, and baked sweet potatoes with a sprinkle of cinnamon. These preparations allowed Sherri the tastes and memories she craved, but in a much healthier way. With meals, she drank tall glasses of ice-cold lemon water.

Sherri needed to protect herself from the possibility of low blood sugar as she began eating less food, so to keep hers stable, we made sure that she had small, high-protein, complex-

carb snacks to eat every 3 or 4 hours. Some diabetes-friendly snacks included shrimp cocktail and crudité with almond butter.

Sherri started the day off with a satisfying, protein-rich breakfast, which she enjoyed. I reminded Sherri that she couldn't skip meals because doing so could cause a drop in blood sugar, a result we did not want. Her blood sugar was consistently monitored. Her diet was basically the same as anyone else's, but her calorie and macronutrient levels were calculated with her specific needs in mind.

Sherri ate fruit (especially citrus and berries); nonstarchy vegetables galore; whole grains (to stabilize her blood sugar and to keep her feeling satiated); and nuts, seeds, eggs, fish, and lean red meat for protein. The meat was treated as an accompaniment, not the main attraction of the meal. In the end, she lost 40 pounds and strutted her new body in a swimsuit, live, on *The View*! She looked divine.

"Dr. Ro has been my nutrition coach since she helped me lose weight in order to get into a bathing suit, live, on *The View*," Sherri says. "It was a crazy thing to do but a lot of fun, and in the process, I lost 40 pounds with her help."

- Whole grains: ½ cup cooked

- Pancakes or waffles: 1 average-size item or a 1-ounce portion

- Popcorn: 3 cups popped, with herbs, spices, or defatted cocoa powder as toppings

- Whole grain breakfast cereal: 1 cup flakes or 1¼ cups puffed

- Rice: ½ cup cooked (1 ounce dry)

- Pasta: ½ cup cooked (2 ounces dry)

WATCH THESE PHASE 3 DIET TRAPS

In Phase 3, continue to cut added sugar as it adds empty calories to your meal plan and is inflammatory to the body. Eat only minimally processed foods if you must include processed foods for convenience. Highly processed foods are a no-no; due to their high-fat, high-calorie, sugar-laden ingredients, many of them contain weight-promoting by-products. Use the time-saving meal prep strategies I've provided throughout the book to prepare nutritious, real food in the shortest possible amount of time. Continue to avoid alcohol or to choose low-calorie options (wine, champagne, light beer, shots of clear liquor) rather than highly sweetened mixed drinks. Doing so will help you meet your weight-loss goals while boosting your health.

The Phase 3 **F-15** Meal Plan

As we've discussed, this third phase of the F-15 Plan includes four servings of protein, three to four servings of vegetables (three on grain days), two servings of fruit, two servings of low-fat dairy, and three servings of fat every day, and one serving of grains three days a week. Although I recommend having protein and vegetables at each meal and snack, the F-15 meal plan gives you the flexibility to allocate your daily servings as you see fit. As in Phases 1 and 2, you may choose to design your own daily menus or use my 15-Day Meal Plans, where I've already done the work for you.

PHASE 3, WEEK 1

Notes about the Meal Plans

- Meal plans include approximately 1,200 to 1,400 calories per day.

- Foods listed in **bold** have recipes in the recipe section.

- Asterisks (*) denote there is a variation in the ingredient amount for that recipe for that specific meal and day.

- Have lemon water with each meal and snack. Lemon water is made with water and the juice of two lemon wedges. Mint lemon water is made by adding 2 tablespoons chopped fresh mint. Basil lemon water is made by adding 2 tablespoons chopped fresh basil. Cucumber lemon water is made by adding 3 to 5 cucumber slices. Or you can mix any combination of these herbs with lemon and/or cucumber for a refreshing drink.

Day 1

MEAL OR SNACK	FOODS	F-15 SERVINGS
Breakfast	Veggie Egg Scramble (1 tablespoon chopped onion, 1 tablespoon chopped fresh basil, ¼ cup sliced mushrooms, 1 cup fresh or frozen spinach, and ¼ cup halved cherry tomatoes mixed with 2 egg whites and 1 whole egg, beaten, and scrambled in 2 teaspoons trans fat–free buttery spread) 1 slice Ezekiel sprouted grain cinnamon raisin bread, toasted, spread with 1 teaspoon trans fat–free buttery spread 1 cup 1% cottage cheese 1 cup green tea 20 ounces lemon water	1 Protein 1 Vegetable 1 Grain 1 Dairy 1 Fat
Morning Snack	½ cup blueberries 20 ounces basil lemon water	1 Fruit
Lunch	1 serving **Lunchtime Turkey Rolls** (page 112) (add 2 teaspoons reduced-fat olive oil mayonnaise) ½ orange 20 ounces basil lemon water	1 Protein 1 Vegetable ½ Fruit 1 Dairy 1 Fat
Afternoon Snack	Turkey Lettuce Wraps (2 ounces roast turkey breast and 1 teaspoon mustard divided and wrapped in 2 lettuce leaves) 20 ounces basil-cucumber lemon water	1 Protein
Dinner	1 serving **Grape Chicken** (page 182) (made with ½ cup grapes) 1 cup kale sautéed in ½ tablespoon extra virgin olive oil and ¼ teaspoon each salt and ground black pepper ½ sweet potato, baked (or microwaved for 7 to 8 minutes), topped with 1 teaspoon trans fat–free buttery spread and a sprinkle of ground cinnamon 20 ounces mint lemon water	1 Protein 1 Vegetable ½ Fruit 1 Fat
Evening Snack	20 ounces lemon water	
	Total for the Day	4 Proteins 3 Vegetables 2 Fruits 1 Grain 2 Dairy 3 Fats

Day 2

MEAL OR SNACK	FOODS	F-15 SERVINGS
Breakfast	1 serving **Black Bean Breakfast Bowl** (page 109) topped with 1 ounce shredded cheddar or Colby cheese 1 cup green tea 20 ounces basil lemon water	1 Protein 1 Vegetable 1 Dairy 1 Fat
Morning Snack	½ cup 1% cottage cheese ½ cup strawberries, sliced 20 ounces lemon water	1 Fruit 1 Dairy
Lunch	Tuna Wrap with Spicy Mayo (4 ounces drained canned water-packed tuna mixed with 1 tablespoon reduced-fat olive oil mayonnaise, ¼ tablespoon Sriracha chili sauce, and ¼ cup chopped spinach divided and wrapped in 6 leaves butterhead lettuce) 1 small apple 20 ounces basil-cucumber lemon water	1 Protein 1 Vegetable 1 Fruit 1 Fat
Afternoon Snack	1 hard-cooked egg 20 ounces mint lemon water	1 Protein
Dinner	1 serving **Asian-Style Beef with Asparagus** (page 185) Tossed Salad (1 cup mixed greens and 1 tomato, chopped, tossed with 2 tablespoons fat-free Italian dressing) 20 ounces basil lemon water with 2 cucumber slices	1 Protein 2 Vegetables 1 Fat
Evening Snack	20 ounces basil lemon water	
	Total for the Day	4 Proteins 4 Vegetables 2 Fruits 2 Dairy 3 Fats

Day 3

MEAL OR SNACK	FOODS	F-15 SERVINGS
Breakfast	1 serving **Savory Tomato Breakfast Bowl** (page 173) 3 scrambled egg whites 2 slices extra-lean Canadian bacon, broiled with 1 spray olive oil cooking spray 1 cup green tea 20 ounces lemon water	1½ Proteins 1 Vegetable 1 Dairy 1 Fat
Morning Snack	20 ounces basil lemon water	
Lunch	Open-Faced Cali Sandwich (1 slice Ezekiel 4:9 sprouted 100% whole grain bread topped with 2 tablespoons Sabra Roasted Red Pepper Hummus; ¼ avocado, thinly sliced; ½ cup grated carrots; ½ cup shredded lettuce; 1 tablespoon fat-free Italian dressing; 1 tomato, sliced; and 2 ounces roast turkey breast) 1 peach 20 ounces basil lemon water	1 Protein 1 Vegetable 1 Fruit 1 Grain 1 Fat
Afternoon Snack	½ cup 1% cottage cheese ½ cup strawberries, sliced 20 ounces basil-cucumber lemon water	1 Fruit 1 Dairy
Dinner	Grilled Salmon, Sautéed Green Beans, and Mixed Green Salad 5 ounces salmon, grilled 1 cup green beans and ½ cup sliced mushrooms sautéed in 1 tablespoon extra virgin olive oil Tossed salad (2 cups mixed greens tossed with 2 tablespoons fat-free Italian dressing) 20 ounces lemon water	1½ Proteins 2 Vegetables 1 Fat
Evening Snack	20 ounces lemon water	
	Total for the Day	4 Proteins 3 Vegetables 2 Fruits 1 Grain 2 Dairy 3 Fats

Day 4

MEAL OR SNACK	FOODS	F-15 SERVINGS
Breakfast	Scrambled Egg Whites, Canadian Bacon, and Yogurt	1 Protein
	2 scrambled egg whites	½ Fruit
	2 ounces extra-lean Canadian bacon, broiled with 1 spray olive oil cooking spray	1½ Dairy
	4 ounces low-fat plain yogurt mixed with 1 tablespoon chopped fresh mint and ⅛ teaspoon ground cinnamon	
	½ cup 1% milk	
	½ apple	
	1 cup green tea	
	20 ounces lemon water	
Morning Snack	Turkey Lettuce Wraps and Egg Whites	1 Protein
	(1 ounce roast turkey breast and 1 teaspoon mustard divided and wrapped in 2 leaves lettuce)	
	2 hard-cooked egg whites	
	20 ounces basil lemon water	
Lunch	1 serving **Open-Faced Shrimp Salad Sandwich** (page 235)	1 Protein
		1½ Vegetables
	Spinach salad (3 cups spinach, ½ tablespoon chopped pecans, and 1 serving **Mandarin Orange Vinaigrette**, page 180)	½ Fruit
		1 Grain
	1 serving **Green Tea–Pom Water Infusion** (page 231)	1 Fat
	20 ounces basil lemon water	
Afternoon Snack	¼ cup 1% cottage cheese	1 Fruit
	½ cup strawberries, sliced	½ Dairy
	20 ounces mint lemon water	
Dinner	Curry Chicken Breast	1 Protein
	(4 ounces boneless, skinless chicken breast sprinkled with lemon juice, salt, ½ tablespoon curry powder, and ½ teaspoon garlic powder and grilled with 1 tablespoon extra virgin olive oil)	1½ Vegetables
		2 Fats
	2 cups kale sautéed in 1 tablespoon extra virgin olive oil	
	½ sweet potato, baked (or microwaved 7 to 8 minutes), sprinkled ⅛ teaspoon ground cinnamon	
	20 ounces lemon water	
Evening Snack	20 ounces lemon water	
Total for the Day		4 Proteins
		3 Vegetables
		2 Fruits
		1 Grain
		2 Dairy
		3 Fats

Day 5

MEAL OR SNACK	FOODS	F-15 SERVINGS
Breakfast	Veggie Egg Scramble	1 Protein
	(2 egg whites and 1 whole egg, beaten; 2 cups spinach; 5 cherry tomatoes, halved; 1 tablespoon chopped onion; ½ tablespoon chopped fresh basil; ¼ cup sliced mushrooms scrambled in 1 tablespoon extra virgin olive oil and ¼ teaspoon each salt and ground black pepper)	1 Vegetable 1 Dairy 1 Fat
	1 slice Ezekiel sprouted grain cinnamon raisin bread, toasted, spread with 1 teaspoon trans fat–free buttery spread	
	½ cup 1% cottage cheese	
	1 cup green tea	
	20 ounces lemon water	
Morning Snack	Spicy Watermelon Chunks	1 Fruit
	(1 cup watermelon chunks sprinkled with ¼ teaspoon chili powder)	
	20 ounces basil lemon water	
Lunch	Smoked Salmon Sushi Roll	1 Protein
	(3 ounces smoked salmon spread with ⅓ tablespoon reduced-fat olive oil mayonnaise mixed with ¼ tablespoon Sriracha chili sauce and rolled into 1 piece nori, topped ¼ avocado, sliced)	1 Fat
	20 ounces basil-cucumber lemon water	
Afternoon Snack	Turkey and Cottage Cheese Wraps	1 Protein
	(3 ounces turkey and ½ cup 1% cottage cheese divided and wrapped in 2 large leaves lettuce)	1 Fruit 1 Dairy
	½ cup strawberries, halved	
	20 ounces mint lemon water	
Dinner	1 serving **Chicken with Tomatoes and Olives** (page 116)	1 Protein
	1 cup green beans, steamed	2 Vegetables 1 Fat
	Tossed Salad (1 cup mixed greens tossed with 1 tablespoon fat-free Italian dressing)	
	20 ounces lemon water	
Evening Snack	20 ounces basil-cucumber lemon water	
	Total for the Day	4 Proteins 3 Vegetables 2 Fruits 2 Dairy 3 Fats

Day 6

MEAL OR SNACK	FOODS	F-15 SERVINGS
Breakfast	1 serving **Savory Tomato Breakfast Bowl** (page 173)	1 Protein
	3 ounces extra-lean Canadian bacon, broiled with 1 spray olive oil cooking spray	1 Vegetable
		1 Dairy
	1 cup green tea	1 Fat
	20 ounces lemon water	
Morning Snack	½ cup strawberries	1 Protein
	4 tablespoons hummus	1 Fruit
	20 ounces lemon water	
Lunch	Roast Beef Lettuce Wraps with Spicy Mayo	1 Protein
	(4 slices deli-style roast beef, 1 slice [1 ounce] low-fat cheddar cheese, 1 tablespoon reduced-fat olive oil mayonnaise mixed with ½ teaspoon Sriracha chili sauce, and 4 thin slices tomato divided and wrapped in 4 leaves lettuce)	1 Vegetable
		1 Fruit
		1 Fat
		1 Dairy
	1 pear	
	20 ounces lemon water	
Afternoon Snack	20 ounces mint lemon water	
Dinner	Baked Haddock, Black Bean Pasta with Tomato and Basil, and Steamed Veggies	1 Protein
	3 ounces haddock, baked or broiled	2 Vegetables
	1 serving **Black Bean Spaghetti with Tomatoes and Basil** (page 184)	1 Fat
	½ cup chopped broccoli florets, steamed	
	Tossed Salad (1 cup mixed greens tossed with 1 tablespoon fat-free Italian dressing)	
	20 ounces lemon water	
Evening Snack	20 ounces basil-cucumber lemon water	
	Total for the Day	4 Proteins
		4 Vegetables
		2 Fruit
		2 Dairy
		3 Fats

Day 7

MEAL OR SNACK	FOODS	F-15 SERVINGS
Breakfast	1 serving **Smoky Salmon Breakfast Scramble** (page 176) ½ cup blueberries 1 cup green tea 20 ounces lemon water	1½ Proteins 1 Vegetable 1 Fruit 1 Fat
Morning Snack	20 ounces mint lemon water	
Lunch	1 serving **Quick-n-Easy Tuna Lunch** (page 178) topped with 1 ounce shredded low-fat cheddar cheese 20 ounces basil lemon water	1½ Proteins 1 Vegetable 1 Dairy
Afternoon Snack	1 piece part-skim mozzarella string cheese 1 small apple 20 ounces basil lemon water with cucumber	1 Dairy 1 Fruit
Dinner	1 serving **Warm Steak Salad** (page 183) 1 serving **Sautéed Brussels Sprouts with Carrots** (page 237) 20 ounces lemon water	1 Protein 2 Vegetables 2 Fats
Evening Snack	20 ounces mint lemon water	
	Total for the Day	4 Proteins 4 Vegetables 2 Fruits 2 Dairy 3 Fats

PHASE 3, WEEK 2

Day 1

MEAL OR SNACK	FOODS	F-15 SERVINGS
Breakfast	1 serving **Yummy Omelet Squares** (page 175) (¼ of the recipe) 3 ounces smoked salmon ½ pink grapefruit 20 ounces basil-cucumber lemon water	1½ Proteins 1 Vegetable 1 Fruit
Morning Snack	20 ounces mint lemon water	
Lunch	1 serving **Turkey and Herbed Cottage Cheese Tomato Wrap** (page 178) 20 ounces lemon water	1 Protein 1 Vegetable 1 Dairy 1 Fat
Afternoon Snack	1 piece part-skim mozzarella string cheese ½ cup strawberries, halved 20 ounces basil-cucumber lemon water	1 Fruit 1 Dairy
Dinner	Broiled Flounder (4 ounces flounder broiled with 5 sprigs chopped fresh dill, juice of 3 lemon wedges, and 1 tablespoon extra virgin olive oil) 1 serving (1 cup) **Red Quinoa and Black Bean Salad** (page 233) 1 serving **Sautéed Spinach** (page 189) 20 ounces lemon water	1½ Proteins 1 Vegetable 1 Grain 2 Fats
Evening Snack	20 ounces mint lemon water	
	Total for the Day	4 Proteins 3 Vegetables 2 Fruits 1 Grain 2 Dairy 3 Fats

Day 2

MEAL OR SNACK	FOODS	F-15 SERVINGS
Breakfast	1 serving **Fat-Burner Smoothie** (page 169) (use ¼ cup pineapple chunks and add ½ cup 1% milk)	2 Proteins ½ Vegetable 1 Fruit 1 Dairy
	1 hard-cooked egg	
	2 ounces extra-lean Canadian bacon, broiled with 1 spray olive oil cooking spray	
	1 cup green tea	
	16 ounces lemon water	
Morning Snack	½ small apple, sliced	1 Fruit 1 Dairy
	½ cup 1% cottage cheese	
	20 ounces basil-cucumber lemon water	
Lunch	Tossed Salad Topped with Tuna	1 Protein 1½ Vegetables 1 Fat
	(2 cups mixed greens; ¼ cup grated carrot; and ½ cup cherry tomatoes, halved, topped with 4 ounces drained canned water-packed tuna and tossed in 1 serving **Dr. Ro's Salad Dressing**, page 181)	
	20 ounces basil-cucumber lemon water	
Afternoon Snack	Stuffed Celery Logs	1 Fat
	(2 stalks celery, cut into thirds, stuffed with 2 table-spoons crunchy almond butter)	
	20 ounces lemon water	
Dinner	1 serving **15-Minute Fish with Cucumber Sauce** (page 113)	1 Protein 2 Vegetables 1 Fat
	1 serving **15-Minute Spaghetti Squash** (page 115), topped with 1½ teaspoons trans fat-free buttery spread	
	1 cup green beans, steamed, topped with 1½ teaspoons trans fat–free buttery spread	
	20 ounces mint lemon water	
Evening Snack	20 ounces mint lemon water	
	Total for the Day	4 Proteins 4 Vegetables 2 Fruits 2 Dairy 3 Fats

Day 3

MEAL OR SNACK	FOODS	F-15 SERVINGS
Breakfast	Veggie Egg Scramble (2 egg whites and 1 whole egg, beaten; ¼ cup sliced mushrooms; 1 tablespoon chopped onion; 1 cup spinach; and ½ cup cherry tomatoes, halved, scrambled in 2 teaspoons trans fat–free buttery spread) 2 slices extra-lean Canadian bacon, broiled with 1 spray olive oil cooking spray 1 slice Ezekiel sprouted grain cinnamon raisin toast topped with 1 teaspoon trans fat–free buttery spread 1 cup 1% cottage cheese 1 cup green tea 20 ounces lemon water	2 Proteins 1 Vegetable 1 Grain 1 Dairy 1 Fat
Morning Snack	Yogurt and Mixed Berries (1 container [5.3 ounces] nonfat plain Greek yogurt mixed with ½ cup blueberries and ½ cup sliced strawberries) 20 ounces basil-cucumber lemon water	2 Fruits 1 Dairy
Lunch	Tossed Salad with Grilled Chicken (4 ounces boneless, skinless chicken breast, grilled and sliced, over 1 cup mixed greens, ½ cup cherry tomatoes, and ½ cup grated carrots tossed in 1 serving **Dr. Ro's Salad Dressing***[made with ½ tablespoon extra virgin olive oil], page 181, and 1 tablespoon fat-free Italian dressing, if desired) 20 ounces mint lemon water	1 Protein 1 Vegetable ½ Fat
Afternoon Snack	20 ounces lemon water	
Dinner	1 serving **Citrus-Ginger Halibut** (page 187) 1 serving **Garlic-Ginger Sautéed Bok Choy** (page 191) 20 ounces basil lemon water	1 Protein 1 Vegetable 1½ Fats
Evening Snack	20 ounces basil-cucumber lemon water	
	Total for the Day	4 Proteins 3 Vegetables 2 Fruits 1 Grain 2 Dairy 3 Fats

Day 4

MEAL OR SNACK	FOODS	F-15 SERVINGS
Breakfast	1 serving **Black Bean Omelet** (page 229) with 1 serving **Tomato-Mango Salsa** (page 230) ½ pink grapefruit 1 cup green tea 20 ounces lemon water	1 Protein ½ Vegetable 1 Fruit 1 Dairy ½ Fat
Morning Snack	1 serving **Zucchini Pizza Wedges** (page 111) 20 ounces basil-cucumber lemon water	1 Protein 1 Vegetable 1 Dairy
Lunch	1 serving **Tropical Shrimp Salad*** (page 232) (use ½ tablespoon reduced-fat olive oil mayonnaise) over tossed salad made with 1 cup mixed greens; 1 Italian tomato, sliced; and 1 serving **Dr. Ro's Salad Dressing** (page 181) 20 ounces mint lemon water	1 Protein ½ Vegetable 1 Fruit 1½ Fats
Afternoon Snack	20 ounces mint lemon water	
Dinner	Baked Salmon (4 ounces salmon baked with ½ teaspoon garlic powder, ¼ teaspoon each salt and ground black pepper, ¼ cup red onion slices, juice of 3 lemon wedges, and 1 tablespoon extra virgin olive oil) 12 spears asparagus, steamed, topped with ½ teaspoon shredded Parmesan cheese 1 small sweet potato, baked (or microwaved for 7 to 8 minutes), topped with 1 teaspoon trans fat–free buttery spread and ¼ teaspoon ground cinnamon 20 ounces lemon water	1 Protein 2 Vegetables 1 Fat
Evening Snack	20 ounces lemon water	
	Total for the Day	4 Proteins 4 Vegetables 2 Fruits 2 Dairy 3 Fats

Day 5

MEAL OR SNACK	FOODS	F-15 SERVINGS
Breakfast	Prosciutto & Grapefruit Breakfast Salad (2 cups mixed greens; ½ cup cucumber slices; 3 hard-cooked egg whites; ½ red grapefruit in sections; 2 slices prosciutto di Parma, torn; and ⅛ cup sliced avocado dressed with ½ tablespoon sesame oil and 1 tablespoon white balsamic vinegar) 1 cup green tea 20 ounces lemon water	2 Proteins 1 Vegetable 1 Fruit 1 Fat
Morning Snack	1 small apple ½ cup 1% cottage cheese 20 ounces mint lemon water	1 Fruit 1 Dairy
Lunch	1 serving **Open-Faced Chicken Sandwich** (page 236) Tossed Salad (2 cups mixed greens tossed with 1 serving **Dr. Ro's Salad Dressing**, page 181) 20 ounces mint lemon water	1 Protein 1 Vegetable 1 Dairy 1 Grain 1 Fat
Afternoon Snack	20 ounces lemon water	
Dinner	1 serving **Black Bean Pasta with Shrimp in Red Curry Sauce** (page 186) ½ cup kale sautéed in ½ tablespoon extra virgin olive oil Tossed Salad (1 cup mixed greens tossed with 2 tablespoons fat-free Italian dressing) 20 ounces lemon water	1 Protein 1 Vegetable 1 Fat
Evening Snack	20 ounces lemon water	
	Total for the Day	4 Proteins 3 Vegetables 2 Fruits 1 Grain 2 Dairy 3 Fats

Day 6

MEAL OR SNACK	FOODS	F-15 SERVINGS
Breakfast	1 serving **Ice Cream Smoothie** (page 168) 3 ounces extra-lean Canadian bacon, broiled with 1 spray olive oil cooking spray 1 cup green tea 20 ounces lemon water	2 Proteins 1 Fruit 1 Dairy
Morning Snack	20 ounces basil lemon water	
Lunch	1 serving **Lunchtime Turkey Rolls** (page 112) Spinach Salad with nuts (2 cups spinach, 1 tablespoon chopped walnuts, and 1 serving **Mandarin Orange Vinaigrette**, page 180) 1 small Granny Smith apple 20 ounces lemon water	1 Protein 2 Vegetables 1 Fruit 1 Dairy 2 Fats
Afternoon Snack	20 ounces mint lemon water	
Dinner	1 serving **Cabbage with Chicken and Apple Sausage** (use 1 cup shredded cabbage*) (page 238) 1 serving **Roasted Potato Medley** (page 234) 20 ounces lemon water	1 Protein 2 Vegetables 1 Fat
Evening Snack	20 ounces basil lemon water	
	Total for the Day	4 Proteins 4 Vegetables 2 Fruits 2 Dairy 3 Fats

Day 7

MEAL OR SNACK	FOODS	F-15 SERVINGS
Breakfast	1 serving **Tuscan Breakfast Salad with Canadian Bacon** (page 108) 1 cup green tea 20 ounces lemon water	2 Proteins 1½ Vegetables 1 Fat
Morning Snack	Celery Sticks Stuffed with Herbed Cottage Cheese (3 large stalks celery stuffed with ½ cup 1% cottage cheese mixed with 5 sprigs dill, chopped) 20 ounces lemon water	1 Vegetable 1 Dairy
Lunch	Turkey Cheeseburger Lettuce Wraps with Spicy Mayo (3-ounce ground turkey patty [93% lean] broiled with ½ tablespoon extra virgin olive oil and topped with 1 slice [1 ounce] low-fat cheddar cheese, ½ tablespoon reduced-fat olive oil mayonnaise mixed with ¼ teaspoon Sriracha chili sauce and ¼ teaspoon each salt and ground black pepper, and 2 tomato slices divided and wrapped in 2 large leaves lettuce) Tossed Salad (1 cup mixed greens tossed with 1 tablespoon fat-free Italian dressing) 1 peach 20 ounces lemon water	1 Protein ½ Vegetable 1 Fruit 1 Dairy 1 Fat
Afternoon Snack	½ cup strawberries 20 ounces mint lemon water	1 Fruit
Dinner	Broiled Steak with Onions and Mushrooms (3 ounces lean beef steak broiled with 2 teaspoons trans fat–free buttery spread and topped with a sauté of 2 cloves garlic, minced; ¼ cup diced mushrooms; and ¼ cup sliced red onion and seasoned with ½ tablespoon Worcestershire sauce, 1 teaspoon reduced-sodium teriyaki sauce, and ¼ teaspoon combined salt and ground black pepper, if desired) 1 cup steamed green beans topped with 1 teaspoon trans fat–free buttery spread 20 ounces lemon water	1 Protein 1 Vegetable 1 Fat
Evening Snack	20 ounces lemon water	
	Total for the Day	4 Proteins 4 Vegetables 2 Fruits 2 Dairy 3 Fats

Day 8

MEAL OR SNACK	FOODS	F-15 SERVINGS
Breakfast	1 serving **Fat-Burner Smoothie** (page 169) (use ¼ cup pineapple and 1 cup spinach and add ½ cup 1% milk*) 1 slice Ezekiel sprouted grain cinnamon raisin bread, toasted, topped with 1 tablespoon almond butter 3 hard-cooked egg whites 1 cup green tea 16 ounces lemon water	2 Proteins ½ Vegetable 1 Fruit 1 Grain 1 Dairy 1 Fat
Morning Snack	10 ounces mint lemon water	
Lunch	Salmon Sushi Roll with Sriracha Mayo and Avocado (3 ounces salmon, grilled or baked, topped with Sriracha mayo [⅓ tablespoon reduced-fat olive oil mayonnaise mixed with 1 teaspoon Sriracha chili sauce]; ¼ avocado, sliced; ¼ cup chopped cucumber; and juice of 1 lemon wedge and rolled in 1 piece nori) Tossed Salad (1 cup mixed greens tossed with 1 tablespoon fat-free Italian dressing) 1 cup watermelon chunks sprinkled with ¼ teaspoon chili powder	1 Protein ½ Vegetable 1 Fruit 1 Fat
Afternoon Snack	Herbed Cottage Cheese (½ cup 1% cottage cheese mixed with 2 teaspoon chopped fresh basil) 20 ounces lemon water	1 Dairy
Dinner	Broiled Flounder with Lemon Butter (4 ounces flounder broiled with 1 tablespoon extra virgin olive oil, juice of ¼ lemon, and ¼ teaspoon each salt and ground black pepper, if desired) 12 spears asparagus, steamed 1 serving **15-Minute Spaghetti Squash** (page 115) 20 ounces lemon water	1 Protein 2 Vegetables 1 Fat
Evening Snack	20 ounces lemon water	
	Total for the Day	4 Proteins 3 Vegetables 2 Fruits 1 Grain 2 Dairy 3 Fats

Grocery List, Phase 3

See list in Phase 1

PHASE 3, WEEK I

MEATS AND FISH

Aidells Organic Chicken and Apple Sausage: 1 package (or from package bought previously)

Beef flank steak: ½ pound

Boneless, skinless chicken breast: ¾ pound

Canadian bacon, extra lean: ¼ pound

Haddock: ¼ pound

Lean turkey salami: 3 ounces

Nori (seaweed sushi wrap): 1 package (typically found in the international foods section of the grocery store)

Roast beef (deli style): ¼ pound

Roast turkey breast (sliced): ¾ pound

Salmon: 1 4 ounces

Salmon lox: 4 ounces

DAIRY

Cheddar or Colby cheese (low fat): 4 ounces

Cottage cheese (1%): 1¾ cups

Feta cheese: ¼ cup

Goat cheese: 1 ounce

Greek yogurt (nonfat, plain): 1 container (5.3 ounces)

Provolone cheese (reduced fat): 1 slice (1 ounce)

String cheese (part-skim mozzarella): 1 (small package)

Yogurt (low fat, plain): 3 containers (4 ounces each)

FRUITS AND VEGETABLES

Apple: 1

Asparagus: ½ cup

Avocados: 2

Bell pepper: 1

Blueberries: 1 cup

Broccoli: 1 cup

Brussels sprouts: 1 cup

Butterhead lettuce: 1 head

Carrots: 2

Cauliflower: 1 cup

Cucumber: 4

Flat-leaf parsley: 1 bunch

Garlic: 5 cloves

Grapes: ½ cup

Green beans: 2¾ cups

Green leaf lettuce: 1 head

Kale: 4 cups

Lemons: 10

Lettuce: 2 leaves

Mixed greens: 2 cups

Mushrooms: 2 cups

Onions: 2

Orange: 1

Peaches: 2

Pear: 1

Pomegranate seeds: ¼ cup

Portobello mushrooms: ½ cup

Red onion: 1

Romaine lettuce: 2½ cups

Scallions: 3

Spinach: 9¼ cups

Strawberries: 3¼ cups

Sweet potatoes: 2

Tangerine: 1

Tomatoes (cherry): 5¼ cups

Tomatoes (Italian or plum): 4

Watermelon: 1 cup

PHASE 3, WEEK 2

MEATS AND FISH

Aidells Organic Sun-Dried Tomato Sausage: 1 package (or from package bought previously)

Boneless, skinless chicken breast: ½ pound

Canadian bacon, extra lean: ½ pound

Flounder: ½ pound

Ground turkey (93% lean): ¼ pound

Haddock: ¼ pound

Halibut: ¼ pound

Lean beef loin steak: ¼ pound

Lean turkey salami: 4 ounces

Nori (dried seaweed sushi wrap): 1 piece

Prosciutto di Parma: 2 slices

Roast turkey breast (sliced): ½ pound

Salmon lox: ¼ pound

Shrimp: ½ pound

Trout: 2 ounces

DAIRY

Almond milk (unsweetened): ½ cup

Cheddar or Colby cheese (low fat): 1 slice (1 ounce)

Cottage cheese (1%): 6 cups

Greek yogurt (nonfat, plain): 2 containers (5.3 ounces each)

Monterey Jack cheese (low fat): 2 ounces

Part-skim (low-fat) mozzarella cheese: 1 slice (1 ounce)

Provolone cheese (reduced fat): 1 slice (1 ounce)

String cheese (part-skim mozzarella): 1 piece

Yogurt (low fat, plain): 3 containers (4 ounces each)

FRUITS AND VEGETABLES

Apples: 2

Asparagus: 3 pounds

Avocados: 3

Banana: 1

Bell peppers: 2

Blueberries: ¼ cup

Bok choy: 1 cup

Butterhead lettuce: 1 head

Cabbage: 1 small head

Carrots: 3

Celery: 1 head

Chives: 1 tablespoon

Cucumber: 4

Fresh cilantro: 1 bunch

Fresh corn: 1 ear

Fresh ginger: 1 piece

Garlic cloves: 4

Grapefruit (pink): 2

Green beans: 2 cups

Green leaf lettuce: 1 head

Kale: 2½ cups

Kiwifruit: 1

Lemons: 10

Lime: 1

Mango: ¾ cup

Mixed greens: 10 cups

Mushrooms: 1 cup

Onion: 1

Orange: 1

Peaches: 2

Pineapple: 1¼ cups

Portobello mushrooms: ½ cup

Purple potatoes: 2 small

Red onion: 1 large

Scallions: 6

Spaghetti squash: 1

Spinach (fresh): 2 pounds

Spinach (frozen): 1 package (10 ounces)

Strawberries: 1 quart

Sweet potatoes: 2 small

Tangerine: 1

Tomatoes (cherry): 2 cups

Tomatoes (Italian or plum): 5

Watermelon: 1 cup

Zucchini: 2

The Phase 3 Recipes

To help you stay on track during Phase 3 of the F-15 Plan, I've created mouthwatering recipes for you, chock-full of delicious, filling foods that fit perfectly into this phase. I love making the earthy, energy-giving Red Quinoa and Black Bean Salad (page 233). It's filling, and marries a barrage of flavors that promise to tantalize your taste buds. The Tropical Shrimp Salad (page 232) is so quick and easy you could almost make it with your eyes closed—but don't! But before you get started, I'd like to call your attention to one of my signature soulful dinners, Cabbage with Chicken and Apple Sausage (page 238). It's dee-lish and so easy to make you don't even have to know how to cook. You're going to love making the dishes in each phase, and I'd love to hear from you and see your food pictures when you make them!

BLACK BEAN OMELET

SERVES 1

1 egg

1 egg white

¼ teaspoon salt

¼ teaspoon ground black pepper

¼ cup drained canned black beans

1 ounce shredded low-fat Monterey Jack cheese

½ tablespoon chopped scallion greens

1 recipe Tomato-Mango Salsa (page 230)

1. In a medium bowl, whisk the egg and egg white, salt, and pepper.

2. In an 8-inch skillet coated with cooking spray over medium heat, cook the egg mixture for 3 minutes, or until set (no stirring).

3. Sprinkle with the beans, cheese, and onion.

4. Loosen the omelet with a spatula and fold in half. Cook for 1 to 2 minutes, or until the cheese melts.

5. Slide the omelet onto a plate. Top with the Tomato-Mango Salsa.

F-15 SERVINGS:	
1	Protein
1	Dairy

NUTRITION INFORMATION:	
Calories:	264
Fat:	12 g
Carbs:	13 g
Protein:	25 g

TOMATO-MANGO SALSA

SERVES 1

¼ cup chopped tomatoes

¼ cup chopped mango

¼ cup chopped red onion

⅛ avocado, chopped

1 tablespoon lemon juice

⅛ teaspoon ground cumin (optional)

In a medium bowl, add the tomatoes, mango, onion, avocado, lemon juice, and cumin, if desired, and mix well.

F-15 SERVINGS:

½	Vegetable
½	Fruit
½	Fat

NUTRITION INFORMATION:

Calories:	89
Fat:	3.5 g
Carbs:	14 g
Protein:	1 g

GREEN TEA–POM WATER INFUSION

SERVES 2

20 ounces water

1 cup green tea brewed from bags (steep 1 green tea bag in hot water for 5 minutes)

½ cup raw pomegranate arils (seeds/juice sacs), crushed

8 leaves fresh mint

In a pitcher, combine the water and green tea. Add the pomegranate and mint. Infuse overnight.

Note: Enjoy infused water as part of your daily caloric budget in 10-ounce portions.

F-15 SERVINGS:

½	Fruit

NUTRITION INFORMATION (PER SERVING):

Calories:	38
Fat:	1 g
Carbs:	8 g
Protein:	1 g

TROPICAL SHRIMP SALAD

SERVES 1

1 ounce lemon juice

1 tablespoon grated lemon peel

⅓ tablespoon reduced-fat olive oil mayonnaise

¼ cup nonfat plain Greek yogurt

4 ounces shrimp, peeled, deveined, cooked, and chopped into bite-size pieces (see note)

¼ cup mango chunks

¼ cup pineapple chunks

¼ cup chopped cucumber

½ tablespoon drained capers, chopped

5 sprigs fresh dill, chopped

1 cup chopped scallion greens

Lettuce leaves

1 sprig dill for garnish

2 thin slices lemon for garnish

1. In a medium bowl, combine the lemon juice, lemon peel, mayonnaise, and yogurt.

2. Fold in the shrimp, mango, pineapple, cucumber, capers, chopped dill, and scallions.

3. Serve on a bed of lettuce. Garnish with the sprig of dill and lemon.

Note: To devein shrimp, cut a small slit down the back of the shrimp and remove the tiny black dorsal line and discard.

F-15 SERVINGS:	
1	Protein
1	Fruit
⅓	Fat
¼	Dairy

NUTRITION INFORMATION:	
Calories:	200
Fat:	3 g
Carbs:	21 g
Protein:	22 g

RED QUINOA AND
BLACK BEAN SALAD

SERVES 8 (SEE NOTE)

1 cup Nature's Earthly Choice
    red quinoa

2 cups water

4 tablespoons fresh lime juice

¼ cup extra virgin olive oil

1 clove garlic, minced

¼ teaspoon salt, plus more to taste

½ teaspoon ground black pepper,
    plus more to taste

½ teaspoon ground cumin

1 can (14 ounces) black beans,
    drained

½ bell pepper, chopped

¼ cup chopped fresh cilantro

2 scallion tops, chopped

1 cup corn kernels

1 avocado, chopped

1 teaspoon hot-pepper sauce
    (optional)

1 small chile pepper, chopped, wear
    plastic gloves when handling
    (optional)

1. In a saucepan, bring the quinoa and water to a boil. Stir, reduce the heat, and simmer for 12 minutes, or until the water is absorbed.

2. Meanwhile, in a small bowl, combine the lime juice, oil, garlic, salt, black pepper, and cumin.

3. When the quinoa finishes cooking, allow it to cool for 5 minutes. Fluff with a fork. Add salt and black pepper to taste.

4. In a large bowl, combine the quinoa, beans, bell pepper, cilantro, scallion, corn, avocado, and hot-pepper sauce and chile pepper, if desired. Add the lime dressing and toss well.

Note: This recipe makes 8 cups; 1 serving is 1 cup.

F-15 SERVINGS:	
1	Grain
¼	Fat
½	Protein

**NUTRITION INFORMATION
(PER SERVING):**

Calories:	139
Fat:	4 g
Carbs:	23 g
Protein:	5 g

ROASTED POTATO MEDLEY

SERVES 2

2 small purple potatoes, cut in half

½ sweet potato, cut in quarters

1 tablespoon extra virgin olive oil

⅛ teaspoon salt

¼ teaspoon ground black pepper

1 teaspoon finely chopped fresh thyme

1 teaspoon finely chopped fresh rosemary

1. Preheat the oven to 400°F.

2. In a medium bowl, toss the potatoes with the oil, salt, pepper, thyme, and rosemary until well coated.

3. Spread the potatoes out on a baking sheet. Roast for 30 to 45 minutes, or until the potatoes are browned and crisp on the outside and tender on the inside (use a fork to pierce potatoes to test for doneness).

F-15 SERVINGS:

1	Vegetable (for Occasional Vegetable days only)
½	Fat

NUTRITION INFORMATION (PER SERVING):

Calories:	143
Fat:	7 g
Carbs:	18 g
Protein:	2 g

OPEN-FACED SHRIMP SALAD SANDWICH

SERVES 1

4 ounces cooked, peeled, and deveined shrimp

¼ cup nonfat plain Greek yogurt

¼ cup chopped peeled cucumber

1 scallion top, thinly sliced

5 sprigs fresh dill, chopped

½ tablespoon drained capers

Grated peel of 1 lemon

Juice of 1 lemon

⅓ tablespoon reduced-fat olive oil mayonnaise

1 slice Ezekiel 4:9 sprouted 100% whole grain bread, toasted

1 leaf lettuce

In a medium bowl, add the shrimp, yogurt, cucumber, scallion, dill, capers, lemon peel, lemon juice, and mayonnaise and mix well. Top the bread with the lettuce leaf and the shrimp salad.

F-15 SERVINGS:

1	Protein
¼	Dairy
1	Grain
⅓	Fat

NUTRITION INFORMATION:

Calories:	221
Fat:	3 g
Carbs:	21 g
Protein:	25 g

**15
MINUTE
RECIPE**

OPEN-FACED CHICKEN SANDWICH

SERVES 1

1 teaspoon mustard

1 slice Ezekiel 4:9 sprouted
100% whole grain bread

2 ounces cooked boneless, skinless
chicken breast, thinly sliced

1 slice (1 ounce) low-fat Monterey
Jack cheese

1. Preheat the oven to broil.

2. Spread the mustard on the bread. Top with the chicken and cheese.
Broil for 2 minutes, or until the cheese is completely melted.

3. Serve immediately.

F-15 SERVINGS:	
1	Protein
1	Dairy
1	Grain

NUTRITION INFORMATION:	
Calories:	233
Fat:	8 g
Carbs:	15 g
Protein:	25 g

SAUTÉED BRUSSELS SPROUTS WITH CARROTS

SERVES 1

1 cup Brussels sprouts, cut into quarters

3 teaspoon trans fat–free buttery spread, divided

1 large carrot, cut into matchsticks

¼ teaspoon salt

¼ teaspoon ground black pepper

Ground cinnamon (optional)

1. Heat a large skillet over medium-high heat for 2 to 3 minutes. Cook the sprouts, 2 teaspoons of the buttery spread, and carrot, stirring frequently, for 2 to 3 minutes.

2. Reduce the heat to medium, cover, and cook for 6 to 7 minutes, or until the veggies are tender.

3. Season with the salt and pepper. Add the remaining 1 teaspoon buttery spread and toss to coat. Sprinkle with the cinnamon, if desired.

F-15 SERVINGS:	
1	Vegetable
1	Fat

NUTRITION INFORMATION:

Calories:	112
Fat:	5 g
Carbs:	15 g
Protein:	4 g

CABBAGE WITH CHICKEN AND APPLE SAUSAGE

SERVES 1

½ tablespoon extra virgin olive oil

1 Aidells Organic Chicken and Apple Sausage, cut into 2"-thick disks on the diagonal

¼ cup chopped red onion

¼ cup chopped yellow or red bell pepper

2 cups shredded cabbage

¼ cup fat-free, low-sodium chicken broth

¼ teaspoon salt

¼ teaspoon ground black pepper

2 tablespoons chopped fresh basil

1 tablespoon chopped fresh thyme

1. In a nonstick skillet over medium-high heat, warm the oil. Cook the sausage and onion for 4 to 5 minutes, or until the onions are opaque and sausage is lightly browned.

2. Add the cabbage and bell pepper and cook for 1 to 2 minutes.

3. Add the broth, salt, black pepper, basil, and thyme. Reduce the heat to low, cover, and simmer for 20 to 30 minutes, or until the cabbage is tender and bright green. Check frequently to ensure the liquid does not completely evaporate.

F-15 SERVINGS:

1	Protein
1½	Vegetables
½	Fat

NUTRITION INFORMATION:

Calories:	305
Fat:	19 g
Carbs:	18 g
Protein:	14 g

Your 15-Minute Moves for Phase 3

You've already got a great collection of 15-Minute Moves from Phase 1 and Phase 2. Here are a few more to add to the mix in Phase 3.

Kickboxing Moves

JAB-CROSS

UPPER BODY, CARDIO

Step 1: Stand with your feet firmly planted on the ground. Place your right foot in front of your left foot and your left foot slightly behind.

Step 2: Keeping your elbows at your sides and your hands in front of your face, punch with your right arm and then pull back to the start.

Step 3: Follow through with a punch with your left arm, and then pull back to the start.

Step 4: Keep your knees soft and pivot your toes on the jab and cross-punch movements to prevent locking your knees in place.

NOTE: Keep the punch or arm extension to 90 percent. Do not lock out your elbows.

Step 5: Reverse the same motion with a left-side stance.

JAB-HOOK FORWARD-STANCE

Step 1: Stand with your feet wider than your hips and soft bent knees, elbows at your sides, hands in front of your face.

Step 2: Starting with your right fist and then alternating between right and left fists, punch right-left and then hook right-left.

Step 3: With your left shoulder slightly dropped and in a slight circular motion, bring your left arm parallel to the floor, punch toward the center of your body, and then return to the start. Repeat on the right side.

Tabata Workout #3

1. Jab-Cross (left foot in front) and alternating front kicks—
   20 seconds of Jab-Cross and 10 seconds of rest;
   20 seconds of alternating front kicks and 10 seconds of rest; repeat the sequence for 4 minutes.

   REST FOR 1 MINUTE.

2. Jab-Cross (right foot in front) and Squats with Front Kicks—20 seconds of Jab-Cross and 10 seconds of rest;
   20 seconds of Squats with Front Kicks and 10 seconds of rest; repeat the sequence for 4 minutes.

   REST FOR 1 MINUTE.

3. Jab-Hook (forward stance) and Squats with Side Kicks—
   20 seconds of Jab-Hook and 10 seconds of rest;
   20 seconds of Squats with Side Kicks and 10 seconds of rest; repeat the sequence for 4 minutes.

   STRETCH. YOU'RE DONE!

   CONGRATS! YOU MADE IT! YOU'RE AWESOME!

SQUATS WITH FRONT KICKS

LOWER BODY (GLUTEAL AND QUADRICEPS MUSCLES)

Step 1: Stand erect, looking straight ahead, with your head and shoulders back. Keep a slight arch in your lower back, your feet hip-width apart, and your arms close to your chest in front of you, elbows bent and hands together with each making a fist.

Step 2: Start to lower your body by pushing your hips back as if to sit on a chair, bending your knees and pushing your body weight into your heels. Remember to keep your chest up and shoulders back while bending from your hips. Always keep a neutral spine for protection.

Step 3: Sit as low as possible (the goal is to have your legs parallel with the floor, but go as low as is comfortable for you; never exceed your comfort level). Sit, with your arms in front of your body, elbows bent, and hands making a fist to assist with balance.

Step 4: Pause at the bottom of the motion before driving through your heels to stand. Keep your knees behind your toes and your weight in your heels for safety and to prevent injury. Give a sharp kick with your right foot on your way up and quickly return to the start position. Repeat the motion, alternating the kick between your left and right foot. **Variation:** For **Squats with Side Kicks**, pause at the bottom and kick to the side, alternating your right and left foot on the way up to the start position.

HIIT Workout #3

TOTAL TIME: 15 MINUTES

1. 1 minute of High Knees (page 124) (beginner: 30 seconds)

2. 30 seconds of Alternating (backward) Lunges (page 128) (beginner: 15 seconds)

REST FOR 30 SECONDS

3. 1 minute of Squats (page 124) (beginner: 30 seconds)

4. 30 seconds of Pushups (page 127) (beginner: 15 seconds)

REST FOR 30 SECONDS

5. 1 minute of Jab-Cross Squat Combo (page 198) (beginner: 30 seconds)

6. 30 seconds of Sumo Squats (page 193)

REST FOR 30 SECONDS

7. 1 minute of Burpees (page 123)

8. 30 seconds of Plank (page 124)

REST FOR 30 SECONDS

9. Repeat the cycle until you've reached your 15-minute mark. Go!

STRETCH. YOU'RE DONE!

CONGRATS! YOU MADE IT! YOU'RE AWESOME!

AMRAP Workout #3

TOTAL TIME: 15 MINUTES

1. Jab-Cross Squat Combo (page 198)—Do 15 reps.

2. Plank Jacks (page 197)—Do 15 reps.

3. Situps (page 123)—Do 15 reps.

4. Sumo Squats (page 193)—Do 15 reps.

5. Rest as needed between rounds. Repeat cycle, doing as many rounds as possible for 15 minutes.

STRETCH. YOU'RE DONE!

CONGRATS! YOU MADE IT! YOU'RE AWESOME!

In the Next Chapter: Maintaining Your Weight Loss

Now that you've learned all about Phase 3 of the F-15 Plan, it's time to talk about maintaining your weight loss. In the next chapter, I'll share my fantastic list of F-15 Lifetime Success Strategies. We'll also discuss some of the things you'll have to look out for based on your body type. Do you have a big belly? A big booty? Either way, I'll help you avoid some common pitfalls. But for now, congratulations on getting this far! You are even stronger than you realize!

Success Story

Jawn Murray

30 pounds lost
10.9 inches lost overall

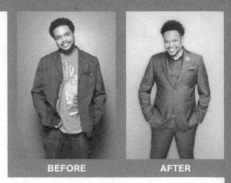

BEFORE **AFTER**

Jawn is a well-known entertainment journalist who travels extensively and was very concerned that his weight gain was making him less appealing on camera. Because he was used to eating on the run and worked late-night hours, he hadn't paid attention to the number of calories he was consuming (sometimes up to 3,500 per day). Jawn knew he couldn't continue down the road he had been traveling.

Jawn's biggest challenge was to learn how to recognize actual serving sizes of foods so that he could cut calories by eating correct portions. He's also a bit of a foodie, which didn't make my job any easier since he likes to "try everything." What he had to learn was the difference between "try" everything (meaning just have a taste, a couple of bites) and "eat it all."

Jawn is insulin-resistant, which means that after eating a meal (especially a meal containing simple sugars, like those found in refined breads, cereals, cookies, and ice cream), his blood sugar and insulin levels remain higher than they should. I started him on Phase 1 of the F-15 Meal Plan to purge his body of all of the junk food he had been consuming and to put his body into a clean and lean state. We fed him vegetables, lean protein, eggs and egg whites, nuts, and seeds, and eliminated bread, grains, and fruit for the first 15 days.

I focused on teaching Jawn about portion sizes, which astonished him.

Like many of my clients who eat out regularly, he had no idea what a normal portion of meat, poultry, fish, or vegetables looked like. He had to be able to eat in restaurants, so we figured out how to make it work for him. He learned to order double green veggies without the starchy side dish and no bread for dinner. At lunch, salads with egg, lean meat, fish, or poultry, and he piled on the veggies.

On Day 15, we decided that he needed more time to adjust to the Phase 1 plan, so we added another 15 days. He had started to lose inches and a few pounds, but I know my clients, and I understood that to introduce anything sweet back into his diet (even fruit) at that point would be a mistake.

When we advanced his meal plan to Phase 2, we stuck with lower-calorie stone fruits (peaches, nectarines, apricots, plums, and cherries), which would have a stabilizing, effect on his blood sugar and insulin levels.

Instead of Jawn just losing the hoped-for 15 pounds, he was so motivated to lose weight that he stuck it out, lost 30 pounds, and took swanky new press photos! "It feels good having my best body back, on *and* off TV," says Jawn.

Chapter 7

SOAR BEYOND THE FINAL 15: RETAIN YOUR WEIGHT LOSS

In the eyes of God all souls are equal.
The same is true of your body; you just have to
own it. Go now and soar!
—Dr. Ro

You've made it! You've reached your weight-loss goal! You've lost that stubborn 15 pounds or 25 pounds or 50 pounds, or maybe you're on your way to losing 100 pounds—God bless you! Thanks to your hard work on the F-15 Plan, you are thinner, healthier, sexier, and in much better shape than you were back when you started. You're eating healthier foods, you've built an exercise habit, and you've learned some ways to reduce stress and take better care of yourself. Your risk of heart disease, diabetes, high blood pressure, and other diseases is most likely lower than it had been. Overall, you're in a much better place than you were in the past. I commend you for your hard work and effort.

The next step is to keep it going! Now here's where it gets tricky. This is the time when you think to yourself, I did it! Now I'll celebrate by going out with the girls for a dessert crawl, or with the fellas for beers or shots. Uh, let me stop you right there. That would be a mistake. It's a slippery slope. Start to do what you used to do and you're sure to start looking like you used to look—before you put in all of that hard work and lost the weight.

The great news is, you did it, but unfortunately, you can't rest on your laurels after losing weight. You can't declare victory and then return to your old habits. During your 45 days (or more) on the F-15

Plan, you've created healthy new habits that can carry you through the rest of your life. Sticking with them is the secret to long-term success. I'm not saying that you can't have a treat once in a while. But unless you want to start packing on pounds again, you'll do best as a weight-loss maintainer if you continue to eat, exercise, and reduce stress the F-15 way.

Each year, millions of people lose weight, but as many as 95 percent of them gain it back within 5 years. That's because they return to their pre-weight-loss habits. You can avoid that fate by continuing to follow the F-15 guidelines long-term. Based on my work with thousands of people who are determined to lose weight and keep it off, I've identified 10 habits that successful long-term weight losers stick to. I call them my F-15 Lifetime Success Strategies. They're not hard to follow; you simply have to decide that this is how you will live your life. You've already been doing most if not all of them during the three phases of my F-15 Plan. Now it's just a matter of extending them into your long-term life plan. In this final chapter of the F-15 Plan, I'll share these strategies with you so that you can stay in your weight-loss sweet spot for the rest of your life.

F-15 Lifetime Success Strategy #1: Eat 15 Servings a Day

In each phase of the F-15 Plan, you've been eating 15 servings of fantastically healthy, fully filling foods. Staying with that 15-serving strategy will allow you to maintain your weight loss for many years to come. Which serving plan should you follow? Here are my guidelines.

If your weight loss is staying steady: Follow the serving plan for Phase 3. This includes four servings of protein, four servings of vegetables (or three on grain days), two servings of fruits, two servings of low-fat dairy, and three servings of fats. And 1 to 3 days a week, have one serving of whole grains instead of one of your vegetable servings. Following Phase 3's serving strategy will allow you to maintain your weight loss.

If your weight inches up by 2 or 3 pounds: Follow the serving plan for Phase 2. This includes four servings of protein, four servings of vegetables, two servings of fruits, two servings of low-fat dairy, and three servings of fats. By leaving out whole grains, you can get back to your target weight quickly. If you want to see results quickly, go straight to Phase 1, your best bet for leaning out body fat.

If your weight goes up by more than 3 pounds: Cycle back to Phase 1 and eat four servings of protein, six servings of vegetables, two servings of low-fat dairy, and three servings of fats. By cutting out fruits and grains and replacing them with lower-calorie everyday vegetables, you rev up your body's fat-burning, muscle-building potential, which helps to bring you back to your target weight quickly.

It's very important for you to nip any weight gain in the bud. If your weight starts going up, take action right away. It's much easier to get back to your goal weight when you've gone up only a couple of pounds, rather than waiting until the scale is way off balance. This is *your* weight loss, *your* body, and *your* future; own it, and do what you have to do to keep yourself where you want to be.

A good way to stay on track is to continue to use your food diary. Back in Chapter 3, I told you all about the benefits of using a food diary to keep track of everything you eat each day. I'm not expecting you to keep a food diary for the rest of your life. But I do recommend that if you find yourself gaining weight instead of maintaining weight loss, going back to your food diary for a few days will help you to get back on track. Keeping a food diary helps you to think more about what you choose to put in your mouth. And it helps to prevent you from practicing mindless eating, one of the biggest obstacles to weight loss. When you write down everything you eat, it helps you be more mindful about what you eat. Keeping a record of what you eat; when you eat it; and the emotions you feel before, during, and after eating can help you to understand the habits and emotions that impact your food choices. So if you find yourself reaching for second helpings of food or sugary, fatty snacks, try reaching for your food diary instead.

F-15 Lifetime Success Strategy #2: Pay Attention to Portion Sizes

It's very easy to become a victim of what I refer to as portion creep. While you're actively losing weight, you pay close attention to portion sizes. But when you move into maintenance mode, you don't focus quite as well on how much goes into a healthy-size portion. Instead of having

Success Story

Amy Seymore

32.4 pounds lost
16.4 inches lost overall

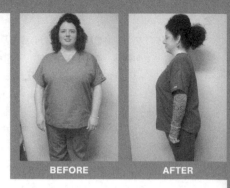

BEFORE **AFTER**

Amy is a dental assistant, wife, and mother who always took pride in her appearance but over time gained weight because her subpar eating habits finally caught up with her. Amy became a master at covering up the extra poundage with stylish, loose-fitting clothing. She was the queen of beach cover-ups, muumuus, and caftans. Her husband was diagnosed with type 2 diabetes. She knew at that point that changing diet and lifestyle was a must for the whole family. She was concerned that the diabetes might lead to other even more serious health problems. It fueled her commitment to help her husband get healthier and became the catalyst that changed both their lives.

Amy was a late-night snacker. Her go-to favorites were Little Debbie cakes, sweet cakes, and potato chips. She had never even considered eating vegetables or fruits for snacks.

To introduce the idea of vegetables and fruits as entrées, side dishes, and snacks, I started with simple swaps. I had Amy try homemade kale chips, which she loved. She used some of her dairy portions of the F-15 Plan to replace potato chips with what I call Cheesy Chips: 1 stick of part-skim mozzarella string cheese cut into thin disklike slices and baked on a baking sheet for 4 minutes, or until brown edges appear on the cheese. As the cheese melts, it browns and starts to resemble potato chips. When the

Cheesy Chips are done and cooled, you simply peel them off and feast on this low-carb, protein-rich snack instead of eating a bag of salty, fatty potato chips. Cheesy Chips are 0 carbs and only 60 calories versus 15 carbs and 160 calories for a small bag of chips. This became a favorite for Amy.

Amy has a busy schedule, so I gave her lots of meal prep tips to help her save time during the day. I had her plan her meals for the week using the F-15 Plan as her guide and prep on weekends, grilling chicken breasts and vegetables, boiling eggs, and making salad dressing to store in the fridge. She would even cut fruit and vegetables to store in clear glass containers in the fridge for later in the week. I recommended that she store them at eye level in the fridge because studies show that adults and teens eat more fruit and vegetables if they can actually see them. With this change, everyone in her family started eating more produce—a positive change for the whole family.

"Losing weight with the F-15 Plan has changed my life, not only physically and mentally, but it gave me more self-confidence," Amy says. "It really gave me a new outlook on life."

a tight handful of nuts, for example, you let your fingers spread a bit, and rather than eating an ounce of almonds, you have an ounce and a half or 2 ounces. And instead of measuring a tablespoon of olive oil into your skillet, you eyeball it and without realizing it, pour in 2 table-spoons. I'm not judging; listen, I do this, too! Portion creep happens to us all! But my point is, if your servings start getting bigger and bigger, you're taking in more and more calories. When portion creep strikes, you're not really eating 15 servings. You're eating 18 or 20 or more servings a day, and that leads to weight gain.

You don't have to be a slave to your measuring spoons or scale. But I do recommend that you stay on top of the correct serving sizes for all foods, especially higher-calorie, higher-fat foods, such as oils, nuts, nut butters, and seeds. Go back to Chapter 3, where I go into detail about portion sizes, and review them every few weeks to make sure you know how much you should be eating. And if you start to gain weight—even just a couple of pounds—take extra care to be sure you're eating the correct portion sizes and not becoming a victim of portion creep.

F-15 Lifetime Success Strategy #3: Exercise Most or All Days of the Week

When you started the F-15 Plan and were just beginning to build an exercise habit, you did one 15-minute routine each day. Then you worked your way up. Now that you've got that habit built, stick with it. The people who have the most success at maintaining weight loss exercise for 30 to 60 minutes per day most or all days of the week. Many do even more exercise than that.

At the very least, get your 15 minutes of high-intensity exercise a day. But if you really want to maintain weight loss, do more than that. I know it may sound intimidating, but the truth is, it's not that hard to exercise for 7 hours a week. It doesn't have to mean spending an hour a day in a gym (yikes, that would bore me to tears, although there are plenty of people who love it). You can hit the 7-hours-a-week mark by working exercise into your everyday activities. Start in small ways—walk the stairs instead of taking the elevator or escalator, park farther away from your destination, get off the bus or train one stop early, that kind of thing. It's amazing how many extra steps you can put into your day with minimal effect on your schedule.

If you're walking, you can also increase your exercise productivity by speeding up. When you first start walking for fitness, it is fine to walk at a leisurely pace. Your goal when you first begin is to build a fitness habit and to become accustomed to fitting 15-minute blocks into your schedule for exercise. But as you become fitter, it makes sense to walk faster. That way, you burn more calories in the same amount of time! Who wouldn't want to do that?

Another way to fit in fitness in everyday life is to make a commitment to active socialization. Think about how much time we spend hanging out with friends and family in very passive ways—many of which involve food and alcohol. We sit at tables in restaurants or at loved ones' houses for hours and hours. Why not go for a walk instead? Rather than sitting at tables or coffee shops or in living rooms consuming vast numbers of calories, I walk with my besties (Simba, Bert, and Ernie—our cocker spaniel and two labs) all the time, and it's amazing how long we walk before realizing how much ground they've all helped me to cover. Get a dog! Adopt one if you can. Seriously! Every time I've lost weight and gotten myself into better shape it started with walking with my dogs. In addition to the exercise they require and insist that you get, they come in a package of unconditional love. There's nothing not to love about that!

When you want to spend time with people you enjoy, plan an active outing, such as a walk, a hike, a cycling trip, or a swim. If a meal is necessary, bring along a picnic made from the recipes in this book. Show people how much fun it can be to be healthy and active. Heck, I even have clients who take their business meetings outdoors (why sit at a table in a stuffy conference room when you can walk outside in the sunshine and discuss business in the fresh air?).

The bottom line is that it's easier than you think to be active; you just have to make a commitment to it and figure out ways to work it into your schedule. Every step you take is a step toward maintaining the weight loss you accomplished on the F-15 Plan.

You already have a nice assortment of 15-Minute Moves from Phases 1, 2, and 3. Now that you're in much better shape than you were when you started, here are a few high-level moves to add to your 15-Minute Moves menu.

JUMP SQUATS

CARDIO, LOWER BODY (GLUTEAL AND QUADRICEPS MUSCLES)

Step 1: Stand erect, looking straight ahead, with your head and shoulders back and a slight arch in your lower back. Stand with your feet hip-distance apart, keeping your arms at your side.

Step 2: Start to lower your body by pushing your hips back as if to sit in a chair, bending your knees and pushing your body weight into your heels. Remember to keep your chest up and shoulders back while bending from your hips, and *always* keep a neutral spine for protection.

Step 3: Sit as low as possible (the goal is to have your legs parallel with the floor, but go as low as is comfortable for you, and *never* exceed your comfort level). As you sit, raise your arms in front of your body or raise them over your head to assist with balance.

Step 4: On the way up from a seated position, jump slightly, just enough to get air under your feet, landing with bent (soft) knees. *Caution:* Never land with locked knees. This can lead to injury. Pause at the bottom of the motion before driving through your heels to stand. Keep your knees behind your toes and your weight in your heels to prevent injury.

ADVANCED TRICEPS DIPS

UPPER BODY, TRICEPS

Step 1: Sit on the edge of a sturdy chair or other elevated surface, placing your palms down beside or under your hips.

Step 2: Bring your body off the chair, keeping your booty close to the chair.

Step 3: Bend at your elbows and lower your body toward the floor. Pause at the bottom before returning to the start.

ADVANCED LEVEL: To add plyometrics (jump training), simply explode from the bottom of the dip to get a little air under your hands and land with soft elbows.

ADVANCED LEVEL PUSHUPS

UPPER BODY, ABS (CORE STRENGTH)

Step 1: Place your toes pointing downward toward the floor, and prepare to push your body up, using your arms and keeping your back flat.

Step 2: Push your body up to the top position, keeping your arms straight. Keep your back flat, never swayed. Keep your head and neck in line with your spine (in a neutral position).

Step 3: Lower your body with your chest almost to the floor, and then push up to the top.

ADVANCED PLANK JACKS

ABS (CORE STRENGTH), UPPER BODY, CARDIO

Step 1: Begin from the top of a pushup position, making sure your hands are below your shoulders.

Step 2: Keep your back flat and your hips pointed toward the floor, and keep your head and neck in line with your spine.

Step 3: Hop your feet out of the plank position and then back in.

BEGINNER LEVEL: First try extending each foot out to the side of plank position, toes still pointed to the floor, and tapping each foot on the floor. Then return one foot at a time back to the center of plank position.

ADVANCED LEVEL: Return both feet at the same time to the center of plank position, which requires a slight jump.

SQUAT WITH ALTERNATING SIDE KICK

CARDIO, UPPER AND LOWER BODY

Step 1: Stand erect, looking straight ahead, with your head and shoulders back and a slight arch in your lower back. Stand with your feet hip-distance apart, keeping your arms at your sides.

Step 2: Start to lower your body by pushing your hips back as if to sit in a chair, bending your knees and pushing your body weight into your heels. Remember to keep your chest up and your shoulders back while bending from your hips, and *always* keep a neutral spine for protection.

Step 3: Sit as low as possible (the goal is to have your legs parallel with the floor, but go only as low as is comfortable for you, *never* exceeding your comfort level). As you sit, raise your arms in front of your body or overhead to assist with balance.

Step 4: Pause at the bottom of the motion before driving through your heels to stand. Keep your knees behind your toes and your weight in your heels to prevent injury. On the way up from the seated position, bring your right knee up and extend your leg to kick to the right side before returning to a squat to repeat on your other leg (squat and kick right, squat and kick left).

F-15 Lifetime Success Strategy #4: Manage Stress

As we discussed in Chapter 4, when your stress reaction gets stuck in the "on" position, you suffer physically and emotionally—and you are likely to gain weight. Research shows that chronic stress contributes to weight gain. And from what I've seen among the people I work with, chronic stress also makes it harder to maintain weight loss. Whether or not you're feeling particularly stressed, I recommend that you continue to spend 15 minutes or more each day focused on relaxation. The relaxation response that can come as a result of stress busters like mindful walking, prayerful meditation, other types of meditation, yoga, and

Success Story

Debra Elrod

91.6 pounds lost
32.7 inches lost overall

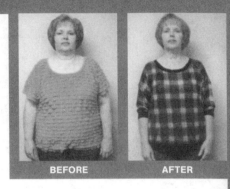

BEFORE   AFTER

Debra has been battling the bulge her whole life. She has never felt comfortable in her own body. Like most overweight and obese people, her self-esteem suffered greatly. She had never really exercised, and her eating habits were consistent with that of a Southern woman from Alabama: oversize portions of fatty fried food. She, like many of my clients, had an out-of-control sweet tooth. She never met a hunk of cake, cookie, or sugar-laden dessert she didn't love.

Debra did not follow a meal schedule. She ate when she thought of it or when she became depressed, bored, or emotionally charged. It is my experience that if a person is 50 or more pounds overweight, there is typically a much deeper emotional cause for the weight. With Debra what mattered most to me was not so much what *she* was eating but rather what was eating *her*. So we dug right into finding the reasons first.

To fix Debra's tendency to rely on food as an emotional crutch, we needed to tease out the feelings that she related to specific foods. I asked her to write down the times she ate when she felt sad, angry, lonely, or just upset, describing her feelings in detail, including the foods she chose to eat in those moments. Often people are not even aware of their feelings or the reasons they have them, let alone their motivations for the behavior they demonstrate when their feelings are connected to food.

We worked on food swaps like air-popped popcorn with Cajun or herb seasoning to replace the fat-laden cheese curls, corn chips, or potato chips she ate when she felt angry or frustrated. When she felt sad, disappointed, or lonely and typically chose ice cream, mashed potatoes, or mac and cheese, we swapped those choices for mashed cauliflower with horseradish, fat-free sour cream, and chives.

Next, we started Debra on Phase 1 and had her alternate between that and Phase 2 for a few months before progressing to Phase 3. She started to see results in the first 15 days, so she was motivated, but to keep her on track and to really change her eating habits, we needed to approach the program this way. To advance her to a maintenance phase of the program before she could make the diet a part of her life might have derailed her progress.

Debra was thrilled with her success: "I never knew what it felt like to just shop in a regular women's store for clothes. Losing the weight has changed my life. I don't worry about being judged because of the way I look anymore. It took me a long time to get here, but now I love this diet and I'm thankful for my new life!"

various other kinds of relaxation techniques help you feel calmer and less frantic and can lead to a measurable decrease in blood pressure, heart rate, breathing rate, stress hormone levels in the blood, and muscle tension. And remember this as you work hard to maintain your weight-loss success: Feeling less anxious and more confident goes a long way toward helping you stay committed to healthy eating, exercise, and other weight-loss maintenance strategies.

F-15 Lifetime Success Strategy #5: Understand Your Problem Areas

Where do you carry your excess weight? Some people are big all over, but most of us have problem areas. The top problem areas are the belly and the butt. That's right—it's very likely that when you put on extra weight, you either get a big belly or a big booty. Which is your problem area? It's a good question to answer, because if you are going to do some extra snacking, you should do it with your problem area in mind.

If you have a big belly, keep it simple: Avoid simple carbohydrates and added sugar. I'm talking soda, candy, and baked goods made with white flour (cake, cookies, brownies, and so on). These kinds of foods can lead to lots of excess belly fat. If you don't believe this when I tell you, take a look at research like this: According to one new study, people who drink sugar-sweetened beverages have more belly fat—also known as visceral fat—than those who don't drink them. Researchers of this 2016 study published in the journal *Circulation* followed more than 1,000 adults, tracked their drinking habits over the course of 6 years, and found that compared with people who never have sugary drinks, those who have at least one sugar-sweetened beverage per day have 27 percent more belly fat. If after reading that you have any doubts about the dangers of sugar-sweetened soft drinks, then nothing will ever convince you to stop drinking them!

Sometimes my clients give up sugary drinks while they're losing weight and then want to start having them again after they reach their weight-loss goals. Don't give in to this sugary temptation! You worked so hard to lose the weight by cutting added sugar from your diet. Remember, if you start to do what you used to do, you begin to look like you used to look, with all of the extra pounds right back where they were before you lost weight on the F-15 Plan. Maintaining weight loss is like having a new suitor, the same thing you did to get 'em, is exactly what you've got to do to keep 'em! As I reported in Chapter 3, studies show Americans could lose about 15 pounds per year if they eliminated sugary beverages. And that's without doing anything else. So think of it this way: If people can lose 15 pounds by eliminating soda, that means you can easily *gain* 15 pounds or more by adding it back into your diet. Pour yourself a glass of nature's champagne—water—or drink unsweetened iced tea instead.

On the other hand, if you've got a big booty, cut or seriously limit your consumption of fatty, salty snacks, which go right to your butt. (Sugary snacks and soft drinks aren't a great idea for you either, but if your belly is flat, your sugar consumption may be under control.) So for the big-bottomed bodies, avoid or limit potato chips, Doritos, corn chips, and the plethora of crunchy, fatty, salty snacks out there. If you've got junk in the trunk, it's likely you're putting lots of junk in your body—junk food, that is. But if you're aware of the fact that your booty is the first place affected when you engage in out-of-control eating, you can take steps to prevent it.

Of the two—big belly or big booty—having a big belly is worse for your health. Studies have found that having belly fat raises your risk of heart disease. There are several reasons for this. Belly fat impacts the kidneys' ability to work properly, which can lead to high blood pressure. As the fat in your belly grows, it surrounds your abdominal organs, such as your kidneys and adrenal glands. People with big bellies also are at an elevated risk for high cholesterol, diabetes, heart attack, and stroke. Belly fat is known to be metabolically active, which means it releases inflammatory agents, hormones, and fatty acids that can have a negative impact on blood cholesterol, blood sugar, and blood pressure.

Even if you are at a normal weight and have excess belly fat, your risk of chronic disease may be elevated. According to Harvard research, normal-weight women with a waist of 35 inches or higher have as much as three times the risk of death from heart disease compared to normal-weight women whose waists are smaller than 35 inches.

If you carry your excess fat in the belly region, please do yourself a favor and cut added sugar from your diet. By losing weight, exercising, and choosing certain fat-burning foods, you can rid your body of harmful, excess belly fat. As you maintain your F-15 weight-loss success, remember to include these fat-burning foods in your diet.

Watermelon: A hydrating fruit rich in lycopene, watermelon can increase your body's levels of arginine, an amino acid that ups the body's fat-burning potential. This juicy red fruit also helps your body build muscle.

Pineapple and papaya: These two tropical fruits contain the enzyme bromelain, which has anti-inflammatory properties and reduces belly fat.

Mint: An herb, yes, but this one goes the extra belly-fat-burning mile. Mint leaves trigger the release of extra bile from the gallbladder, which is important because it helps the body to digest fat. For a quick remedy to belly bloat (maybe you want to ease into that little form-fitting black dress?), add 10 crushed mint leaves to 2 to 4 cups of roasted dandelion tea every day.

Dandelion root: I like roasted dandelion root tea to beat belly fat. Dandelion root increases liver function, which flushes toxins and excess water from the belly area and in turn gives you a flatter tummy.

F-15 Lifetime Success Strategy #6: Plan for Mistakes— Because Life Happens!

Let's face it: No matter how hard you try, how many promises you make to yourself, or how seriously committed you are to the F-15 Plan and your own personal health journey, mistakes happen because we humans are fallible. You might down an entire family-size bag of potato chips when you have a romantic disappointment. You could be one of those people who eat a whole rack of baby-back ribs when your team is winning the big game. After trying "just a bite" of chocolate cake at an amazing restaurant, you might go ahead and have the entire slice because it is simply one of the best things you've ever tasted in your life.

If you slip up while on this diet, relax. It's (hopefully) one meal and nobody died—a barometer we use to determine how serious things really are in my family when life gets crazy. Hey, I'm married to an aesthetic medicine physician who worked over 20 years as an ER doc, what can I say? Here's the thing. We all make mistakes. The secret to dealing with mistakes is to acknowledge them, forgive yourself, and then get right back on track. It won't help to beat yourself up—do that, and you'll just end up making more mistakes as you wallow in self-pity. Instead, acknowledge that mistakes are part of being human; we all make them. Then, once you acknowledge that you slipped off the wagon, forgive yourself and move on! That way, you limit the damage done by making just one mistake. Face it, no one likes starting over after a long course of hard work. Why set yourself up for that disappointment?

And remember: Sometimes physical hunger has nothing at all to do with your desire to eat. Food cravings can be a sign of something completely different from emotional or physical hunger; they can actually be your body's way of telling you you're thirsty or tired or that your muscles need moving. Next time you have a craving, see if a tall glass of ice water, a nap, or 10 minutes of exercise chase it away. You may be surprised to see your hunger disappear without a single bite of food.

There may come a time when you won't want to deny yourself a food because sometimes we just need a little relief. Life happens, and sometimes you just need a cocktail or to dive into a boat of ice cream to feel better for the moment. Here's an example of that happening in my life. Recently, my beloved cocker spaniel, Simba, was hit by a truck and very badly injured. Now, Simba isn't just any dog. He is the apple of my eye, a dog who has brought me through some devastating life events, who has loved me unconditionally for nearly a decade!

Simba's accident was devastating to me (he very nearly died and experienced traumatic head injuries and a concussion). When he came home from the hospital, Simba needed round-the-clock care and twice-daily physical therapy, which I happily undertook. He also got up multiple times during the night, leaving me exhausted the next day. One evening in the middle of this, I opened a bottle of champagne and poured myself a big glass. At the time, I was following my own advice—staying away from sugar, alcohol, and fatty foods—so I could look my best for the cover shoot for this book. But I was physically and emotionally exhausted, and I simply needed an escape, which the bubbly provided at that moment.

That night, there's no question about it: I deserved a drink or two, and I don't apologize for having had it. But the next day I got right back on the horse and returned to following the F-15 Plan. Life must go on. We have to plan for mistakes and failure and then just keep on going in order to achieve and maintain our goals.

Simba update: The vets had given up on him and said his condition would not improve. He had lost control of his faculties and was unable to walk, and because of the brain swelling he endured, he moved only in a circle to the left. By God's grace, Simba is now running, not walking, and is doing everything he did before the accident, except that he continues to limp and must run using three legs until his broken bones in one paw heal. God is amazing, and Simba is a champion!

F-15 Lifetime Success Strategy #7: Weigh Yourself Once a Week

I don't want you to become obsessed with the numbers on a scale. After all, good health depends on so much more than just how many pounds you weigh. But in order to nip any weight gain in the bud, it's important to stay on top of the numbers. By weighing yourself every week, you can jump into action the minute you notice the pounds coming back. It's easy to lose a pound or two but much, much harder to lose 10 or 20 pounds. So jump on the scale weekly, and if the numbers start going up even a little, go back to Phase 1 and then to Phase 2 and stop them in their tracks. When you get on the scale and like what you see, consider giving yourself some kind of a reward. You deserve it! Choose nonfood rewards, of course (you certainly can't pat yourself on the back for a weight-loss success with a brownie or a cupcake; that would be absurd!). When you set and achieve a goal, give yourself something special—anything from

BETTER THAN POTATO CHIPS

I have yet to meet the person who doesn't enjoy a good potato chip, and for good reason. It is the perfect combination of a salty, buttery flavor with a crunchy bite that satisfies. But a single-serving bag of potato chips has 15 grams of carbs and 160 calories, and the truth is, most people don't eat just one—bag. Fortunately, the same cheesy chip recipe that I gave earlier (see Amy Seymore's story on page 248) may satisfy the chip lover in you, too.

a new pair of earrings for a smaller goal to a few days of vacation for meeting a big goal! Take it from me: Rewards work!

F-15 Lifetime Success Strategy #8: Be the Last One at the Table to Eat

You may have experienced this before. You're having dinner with a racy eater who's finished her plate before you could get through the appetizer. Well, keeping pace with fast eaters when dining with others will keep weight on you! That's right, it turns out that when dining with others who eat like speed racers, you are unconsciously prompted to keep up with the fastest eater at the table, shoveling in extra calories, too. It takes 20 minutes for the brain to receive and process the signal from the stomach that you're full. Eating slowly gives your stomach and brain time to realistically register the amount of food and calories that you have consumed.

You have a much better chance of operating from a position of strength and self-control if you slow down the pace of eating your meals. That's why I recommend being the last one at the table to start eating. Rest your fork or spoon between bites, and take the time to chew each bite of food 15 times. These small but helpful tips will net you a big payoff!

F-15 Lifetime Success Strategy #9: Create a Community of Like-Minded People

This is a really important strategy for long-term weight-loss success. When you're maintaining weight loss, it's much easier to stay on track when you're surrounded by people who support you and who share your commitment to healthful eating, fitness, and stress management. I'm sure you've seen this yourself many times. You know what it's like to have that friend who pushes you to eat too much or that aunt who pouts when you don't have seconds at her dinner table. And you know how much easier it is when you are socializing with the friend who would rather go for a walk than eat a heavy meal or the sister-in-law who serves fresh fruit for dessert rather than a huge cake with buttercream frosting.

I'm not telling you to abandon your family or to stop spending time with your friends. But I am encouraging you to, as much as possible, spend time with people who support your lifestyle choices. It's just so much easier when you are not forced to tussle with people about food and exercise.

As for the people who don't support you and perhaps are even trying to sabotage your success, take a look at why they may feel that way. Are they jealous of you? Are they afraid of losing you? Do they wish they could have the success you're having but are afraid or unsure of how to do it? I have a number of clients whose spouses became jealous, angry, or even verbally abusive when they started to lose weight. Most of these spouses were overweight also, and they were afraid that if their spouses lost the weight, their love would be threatened. If this happens to you, talk gently with your spouse about his or her hopes and fears. If necessary, make an appointment with a marital counselor or a trusted pastor. Often these problems can be cleared up with loving communication. You may even be able to convince your partner to start following the F-15 Plan, too!

Weight-loss support groups can also be a good way to create a community of support. These groups provide an opportunity for you to receive (and give) encouragement, tips, and advice. Some groups even gather in each other's homes periodically to cook and freeze healthy meals to share. Check out local churches, health clubs, and community centers to see if you can find a weight-loss support group in your area. You can even start your own group by networking with family and friends. Or check out the various online support groups. Having people who are in your corner really can make a difference.

F-15 Lifetime Success Strategy #10: Focus on Life, Rather Than Food

To understand what I'm thinking about here, rewind to the last time you got together with a big crowd of family and friends. Maybe it was Christmas or someone's birthday or a retirement party or a Fourth of July picnic. Whatever it was, use your visualization skills and picture it in your mind: Whatever the event, there were lots of people and lots of food. Now think back to what you focused on during the event. Were you by the buffet table, making sure you got seconds and thirds of the tastiest dishes? Or were you focused on the people, laughing and sharing stories with friends and family? My point is this: Too often at parties and in life, we are so focused on what we're going to put in our mouths that we miss the most important gift there is—actually *living* and spending time with those whom we love. In other words, we've become so food-obsessed that we think more about our stomachs than we think about life around us.

What I want you to do as you maintain the success you achieved with the F-15 Plan is to start thinking less about food and more about living life to its fullest. Life is the biggest gift we'll ever receive, and too often we lose sight of that because we're sidetracked by less-important things. I encourage you to use the mindfulness skills we reviewed earlier in this book to focus on living a happier, more fulfilling, more satisfying life. Let food take a backseat to the more important things in this world. When you're at a party, it's fine to enjoy the meal you're given, but that will never be as important as the time you get to spend with your loved ones. Try always to remain mindful of what truly matters.

Join the Final 15 Movement!

Get the support you need; share your story, photos, progress, pitfalls; and allow me to continue to support you on your Final 15 journey. I want this to be a successful and enjoyable experience for you and will, as I promised in earlier pages, be there to support you throughout the process. Share your experience with family, friends, coworkers, and your entire network on social media. Encourage them to join us in this Final 15 movement! Together we can make a difference in reversing America's obesity epidemic. Ask them to buy the book and get started on what could be the best thing that ever happened to them...the result of good health, finally, and a happy life.

I urge you and your network to connect with me here:

Your private F-15 Facebook group:

facebook.com/groups/DrRoFinal15/

Success Story

Drew Dale

29.4 pounds lost

9.5 inches lost overall

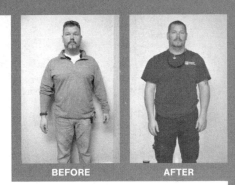

BEFORE   **AFTER**

Drew, a fireman who had a (weight-loss) fire of his own to put out, gained weight when he ditched his snuff-dipping habit and started to rely on a steady diet of fast-food burgers, fries, and sugary drinks to replace the tobacco. First he noticed his pants were fitting a bit more snugly than they had been in previous years. Then his energy began to wane. He knew that he had to lose the weight in order to adequately perform the duties of his job. To add insult to injury, his eating habits were sporadic because he never knew when he'd eat his next meal. Even when he and his coworkers prepared meals at the fire station, the meals weren't the healthiest.

To help Drew, I knew that first we needed to get his taste buds back on track. He had practically forgotten how good real food actually tasted since he had masked the taste with dipping tobacco and eating mostly high-fat foods. He ate hardly any fresh fruits or vegetables except iceberg lettuce in the occasional side salad. To get Drew back to basics, we incorporated copious amounts of vegetables and then fruit in his diet. He snacked on them and included them in all of his meals.

Next we had to address the big, red elephant in the room. Drew spent most of his working hours at the fire station or on the scene, fighting fires. What he

ate with his coworkers counted toward his daily calorie budget and nutrient consumption, so we needed to make reasonable changes there, too.

I taught Drew how to modify recipes and to make simple swaps, such as brown rice or quinoa spaghetti with turkey meatballs, to replace the refined pasta and the fatty sausage, full-fat ground beef, and sugary sauce he often ate at the firehouse before. Drew and I also focused on meal prep for his days off and for his buddies at the firehouse. If a fire broke out in the midst of a healthy meal, they had to leave the meal and go quickly! So we focused on grab-n-go snacks and small meals that he could take with him, such as hard-cooked eggs, chicken and turkey lettuce wraps, veggies packed in resealable plastic bags with a squeeze of hummus. Drew even prepped batches of oatmeal ahead of time that he could freeze and microwave at the firehouse. Now, not only is Drew off tobacco, but he is healthier and leaner and has energy to burn.

"What I like about Dr. Ro's F-15 Plan is that it helped me lose weight and get in shape, and she taught me how to eat, too," says Drew.

E-mail me in the private F-15 Facebook group:

DrRoFinal15@groups.facebook.com

Join my newsletter at:

https://everythingro.com

Like and join my Dr. Ro Facebook page for daily inspiration and health tips:

facebook.com/1drro

Twitter:

@everythingro

Instagram:

@everythingro

Contact me at https://everythingro.com if you'd like to learn more about personal coaching or programs that provide coaching, online support groups, and personalized meal plans. I am here to help you!

ACKNOWLEDGMENTS

A kind and grateful heart need know no bounds nor should it be hidden. To that end, there are a few skilled and loving spirits who have generously given of themselves and enriched my great life and this work. I'd like the world to know your names because you mean so much to me.

To my patients at Dr. Riggins MASC and to the clients of my private coaching practice, I offer abundant thanks for your trust in me, for agreeing to be a part of this work, and for so generously sharing your stories for the benefit of others. May you continue to find your path to a lifetime of joy and maintaining a healthy weight!

To my MASC team, your love and support humbles me. Together we are changing lives, one meal at a time!

To Dr. Murray Riggins, you are both the greatest healer I know and the gold standard for husbands. Twice now you have supported me through the long and arduous process of writing a book, a feat not easy for most. This one was no exception. I love you and owe you lots! "Soon as I get my money right!"

To my agent, Sarah Passick, at Sterling Lord Literistic, you are literally one of the hardest-working, brightest women I know. For going to bat for me, fighting for your client as you would yourself, and for the sheer brilliance of an iron will encased in kindness, I sincerely thank you! We make a great pair.

To an editor among editors whom I now call a friend, Porscha Burke, you, with your brilliant self, believed in me when no one else would. You and you alone said yes when the power of God came to enlist a change agent to be my beacon. Even my love of words eludes my senses to thank you sufficiently.

To my Rodale team, in a way that gives new meaning to "collaboration," you are a well of support for me and for this work. Thank you. Every one of you, stellar!

To Alice Lesch Kelly, abundant thanks for your keen eye and dutiful assistance in bringing this work to fruition.

To Tiffany Jacobs, my Alabama personal trainer, you get me! Thanks for your brilliance and for insisting that a part of me (mostly my fat) die a little each time we meet so that I might live on in a stronger, more fit, and toned body—someday!

To Dr. Mehmet Oz, I could not have imagined that all those years before *The Dr. Oz Show,* as you stood on the stage of the Governor and First Lady's conference and I followed, that we would be here. Thank you for your support and for providing the platform for me to serve a world in need. It means more than you know.

To Stacey Rader, you are a brilliant producer and kind soul. It is a joy to know and work with you.

To Geoff Rosen, a television force, thank you for your support. We make great TV together!

To Jawn Murray, a client and a friend, I'm eternally grateful for your unwavering love and support. I adore you.

To Sherri Shepherd, a hard-working mother, a fearless and talented actress, and a self-described "Jesus freak," thank you for your support, your open heart, and your willingness to be a part of this work.

To my family: Thelma Quick, Pearline and John Singletary, Gloria Wiggs, Cheryl Quick, Charnelle and Corey Anderson, Dante Quick, Ameyon "JoJo" Quick, Antoinette Junious, Dee and Willie Jolley, and Mary Rullow, thank you for your continued love, prayers, and support. No matter how far this trek may take me, I will always have all of you to keep my head level and my heart open.

Gloria, my big Sis, you are a force of sisterhood and friendship. You have always challenged me to master and captain my fate. A special thank you!

To makeup genius and friend Merrell Hollis, thank you for giving me a good face for the jacket of this book and always. You know every line and blemish intimately and help me to show up fully as myself, beautifully.

To Johnjalene Woods of Favor Hair Studio, thank you for putting your styling and natural hair care gifts to work for the health of my mane regularly and for this book cover. You, with your beautiful soul, are an inspiration.

To Virginia State University, my undergraduate alma mater and the base of preparation that allowed me to soar, a sincere and heartfelt thank you.

To Dr. Allan Johnson, a mentor and friend, and to the faculty of the department of nutritional sciences at Howard University, who nurtured and poured into me the best of what I've become as a nutritionist, a sincere thank you to each who's been a willing participant and inspirational source. I arrived at Howard University as Rovenia Brock but left as Dr. Ro, a most fruitful and fulfilling stop on my journey to say the least. To you, I am most grateful.

To you all, may you experience the love, peace, and fulfillment that you have so graciously spawned in me!

BIBLIOGRAPHY

Introduction

Magkos, Faidon, Gemma Fraterrigo, Jun Yoshino, et al., "Effects of Moderate and Subsequent Progressive Weight Loss on Metabolic Function and Adipose Tissue Biology in Humans with Obesity," *Cell Metabolism* 23, no. 4 (2016): 591–601.

Chapter I

"2014 National Diabetes Statistics Report," Centers for Disease Control and Prevention, last modified May 15, 2015, cdc.gov/diabetes/data/statistics/2014statisticsreport.html.

"Basics about Diabetes," Centers for Disease Control and Prevention, last modified March 31, 2015, cdc.gov/diabetes/basics/diabetes.html.

Berg, Christina, and Helene Berteus Forslund, "The Influence of Portion Size and Timing of Meals on Weight Balance and Obesity," *Current Obesity Reports* 4, no. 1 (2015): 11–18.

"CDC Prediabetes Screening Test," Centers for Disease Control and Prevention, accessed May 24, 2016, cdc.gov/diabetes/prevention/pdf/prediabetestest.pdf.

"Diagnosis of Diabetes and Prediabetes," National Institute of Diabetes and Digestive and Kidney Diseases, June 2014, niddk.nih.gov/health-information/health-topics/Diabetes/diagnosis-diabetes-prediabetes/Pages/index.aspx.

"Heart Disease and Obesity," American Heart Association, last modified February 2014, www.heart.org/HEARTORG/GettingHealthy/WeightManagement/Obesity/Obesity-Information_UCM_307908_Article.jsp#.Vo17MVn_spA.

"Heart Disease Fact Sheet," Centers for Disease Control and Prevention, last modified November 30, 2015, cdc.gov/dhdsp/data_statistics/fact_sheets/fs_heart_disease.htm.

"Large Portion Sizes Contribute to U.S. Obesity Problem," National Heart, Lung, and Blood Institute, accessed May 24, 2016, www.nhlbi.nih.gov/health/educational/wecan/news-events/matte1.htm.

"Obesity and Cancer Risk," National Cancer Institute, last modified January 3, 2012, cancer.gov/about-cancer/causes-prevention/risk/obesity/obesity-fact-sheet.

"Overweight and Obesity Statistics," National Institute of Diabetes and Digestive and Kidney Diseases, October 2012, niddk.nih.gov/health-information/health-statistics/Pages/overweight-obesity-statistics.aspx.

"Prediabetes: Could It Be You?," Centers for Disease Control and Prevention, accessed May 24, 2016, cdc.gov/diabetes/pubs/statsreport14/prediabetes-infographic.pdf.

"The Genetics of Diabetes," American Diabetes Association, last modified May 20, 2014, diabetes.org/diabetes-basics/genetics-of-diabetes.html.

"The Impact of Obesity on Your Body and Health," American Society for Metabolic and Bariatric Surgery, accessed May 24, 2016, asmbs.org/patients/impact-of-obesity.

Chapter 2

Anton, Stephen D., Jacqueline Gallagher, Vincent J. Carey, et al., "Diet Type and Changes in Food Cravings following Weight Loss: Findings from the POUNDS LOST Trial," *Eating Weight Disorders* 17, no. 2 (2012): e101–e108.

Cheren, Mark, Mary Foushi, Ester Helga Gudmundsdotter, et al., "Physical Craving and Food Addiction," The Food Addiction Institute, accessed May 24, 2016, foodaddictioninstitute.org/FAI-DOCS/Physical-Craving-and-Food-Addiction.pdf.

Fesler, Katie, "The Craving Brain," *Tufts Now*, February 11, 2014, now.tufts.edu/articles/craving-brain.

Kemps, Eva, Marika Tiggemann, and Sarah Bettany, "Non-Food Odorants Reduce Chocolate Cravings," *Appetite* 58, no. 3 (2012): 1087–90.

Meule, Adrian, and Julia M. Hormes, "Chocolate Versions of the Food Cravings Questionnaires. Associations with Chocolate Exposure-Induced Salivary Flow and Ad Libitum Chocolate Consumption," *Appetite* 91 (2015): 256–65.

Pollan, Michael, *Cooked: A Natural History of Transformation*, New York: Penguin, 2014.

Skorka-Brown, Jessica, Jackie Andrade, and Jon May, "Playing Tetris Reduces the Strength, Frequency, and Vividness of Naturally Occurring Cravings," *Appetite* 76, (2014): 161–65.

Van Kleef, Ellen, Mitsuru Shimizu, and Brian Wansink, "Just a Bite: Considerably Smaller Snack Portions Satisfy Delayed Hunger and Craving," *Journal of Food Quality and Preference* 27, no. 1 (2013): 96–100.

Chapter 3

Au, N., G. Marsden, D. Mortimer, and P. K. Lorgelly, "The Cost-Effectiveness of Shopping to a Pre-Determined Grocery List to Reduce Overweight and Obesity," *Nutrition & Diabetes* 3 (2013): e77, doi:10.1038/nutd.2013.18.

"Eggs and Heart Disease," Harvard T.H. Chan School of Public Health, accessed May 24, 2016, hsph.harvard.edu/nutritionsource/eggs/.

Garaulet, Marta, Purificación Gómez-Abellán, Juan J. Alburquerque-Béjar, et al., "Timing of Food Intake Predicts Weight Loss Effectiveness," *International Journal of Obesity* 37, no. 4 (April 2013): 604–11.

Hollis, Jack F., Christina M. Gullion, Victor J. Stevens, et al., "Weight Loss during the Intensive Intervention Phase of the Weight Loss Maintenance Trial," *American Journal of Preventive Medicine*, 35, no. 2 (August 2008): 118–26.

Imamura, Fumiaki, Laura O'Connor, Zheng Ye, et al., "Consumption of Sugar Sweetened Beverages, Artificially Sweetened Beverages, and Fruit Juice and Incidence of Type 2 Diabetes: Systematic Review, Meta-Analysis, and Estimation of Population Attributable Fraction," *BMJ* 351 (2015): h3576, doi:10.1136/bmj.h3576.

"Insufficient Sleep Is a Public Health Problem," Centers for Disease Control and Prevention, last modified September 3, 2015, cdc.gov/features/dssleep/.

Just, David R., and Brian Wansink, "One Man's Tall Is Another Man's Small: How the Framing of Portion Size Influences Food Choice," *Health Economics* 23, no. 7 (July 2014): 776–791.

"Just Enough for You: About Portion Size," National Institute of Diabetes and Digestive and Kidney Diseases, June 2012, niddk.nih.gov/health-information /health-topics/weight-control/just-enough/Pages/just-enough-for-you.aspx.

Kumar, Gayathri S., Liping Pan, Sohyun Park, Seung Hee Lee-Kwan, Stephen Onufrak, and Heidi M. Blanck, "Sugar-Sweetened Beverage Consumption among Adults—18 States, 2012," *Morbidity and Mortality Weekly Report* 63, no. 32 (August 15, 2014): 686–90.

"National Weight Control Registry Facts," National Weight Control Registry, accessed March 24, 2016, nwcr.ws/Research/default.htm.

"Nuts for the Heart," Harvard T.H. Chan School of Public Health, accessed May 24, 2016, hsph.harvard.edu/nutritionsource/nuts-for-the-heart/.

Pollan, Michael, *The Omnivore's Dilemma: A Natural History of Four Meals*, New York: Penguin, 2007.

"Portion Size versus Serving Size," American Heart Association, accessed May 24, 2016, www.heart.org/HEARTORG/GettingHealthy/ HealthierKids/HowtoMakeaHealthyHome/Portion-Size-Versus-Serving -Size_UCM_304051_Article.jsp#.

Wansink, Brian, and Craig Wansink, "The Largest Last Supper: Depictions of Food Portions and Plate Size Increased over the Millennium," *International Journal of Obesity* 34 (2010): 943–44.

"What Is Sleep Apnea?," National Heart, Lung, and Blood Institute, last modified July 10, 2012, www.nhlbi.nih.gov/health/health-topics/topics /sleepapnea.

"Work Schedules: Shift Work and Long Hours," Centers for Disease Control and Prevention, last modified August 5, 2015, cdc.gov/niosh/topics/workschedules/.

Zmuda, Natalie, "Bottoms Up: A Look at America's Drinking Habits," *Advertising Age*, June 27, 2011, adage.com/article/news/consumers-drink-soft-drinks-water-beer/228422/.

Chapter 4

"Fact Sheet on Stress," National Institute of Mental Health, accessed May 24, 2016, nimh.nih.gov/health/publications/stress/index.shtml.

Leidy, Heather J., Peter M. Clifton, Arne Astrup, et al., "The Role of Protein in Weight Loss and Maintenance," *American Journal of Clinical Nutrition* 101, no. 6 (June 2015): 1320S–29S.

"National Weight Control Registry Facts," National Weight Control Registry, accessed March 24, 2016, nwcr.ws/Research/default.htm.

Pot, G. K., A. M. Stephen, C. C. Dahm, et al., "Dietary Patterns Derived with Multiple Methods from Food Diaries and Breast Cancer Risk in the UK Dietary Cohort Consortium," *European Journal of Clinical Nutrition* 68, no. 12 (December 2014): 1353–58.

Weir, Kirsten, "The Exercise Effect," *Monitor on Psychology* 42, no. 11 (December 2011): 48.

Young, Simon N., "How to Increase Serotonin in the Human Brain without Drugs," *Journal of Psychiatry and Neuroscience* 32, no. 6 (November 2007): 394–99.

Zhang, Yuan, Shiwu Lia, William Donelan, et al., "Angiopoietin-Like Protein 8 (Betatrophin) Is a Stress-Response Protein That Down-Regulates Expression of Adipocyte Triglyceride Lipase," *BBA Molecular and Cell Biology of Lipids* 1861, no. 2 (February 2016): 130–37.

Chapter 5

"AICR's Foods That Fight Cancer," American Institute of Cancer Research, accessed May 24, 2016, aicr.org/foods-that-fight-cancer/.

Food and Nutrition Board, *Dietary Reference Intakes for Energy, Carbohydrate, Fiber, Fat, Fatty Acids, Cholesterol, Protein, and Amino Acids*, Washington, DC: The National Academies Press, 2005.

Hanson, Corrine, Elizabeth Lyden, Stephen Rennard, et al., "The Relationship between Dietary Fiber Intake and Lung Function in the National Health and Nutrition Examination Surveys," *Annals of the American Thoracic Society* 13, no. 5 (2016): 643–50.

"The Benefits of Beans and Legumes," American Heart Association, last modified January 2015, heart.org/HEARTORG/HealthyLiving/HealthyEating/SimpleCookingwithHeart/The-Benefits-of-Beans-and-Legumes_UCM_430105_Article.jsp#.VsixEdD_spA.

Chapter 6

Wu, Hongyu, Alan J. Flint, Qibin Qi, et al., "Association between Dietary Whole Grain Intake and Risk of Mortality: Two Large Prospective Studies in U.S. Men and Women," *JAMA Internal Medicine* 175, no. 3 (2015): 373–84.

Chapter 7

Chandra, Alvin, Ian J. Neeland, Jarett D. Berry, et al., "The Relationship of Body Mass and Fat Distribution with Incident Hypertension," *Journal of the American College of Cardiology* 64, no. 10 (2014): 997–1002.

"Study: Belly Fat May Lead to High Blood Pressure by Affecting Kidneys" American Heart Association, October 22, 2014, blog.heart.org/study-belly-fat-may-lead-to-high-blood-pressure-by-affecting-kidneys/.

"Waist Size Matters," Harvard T.H. Chan School of Public Health, accessed May 24, 2016, hsph.harvard.edu/obesity-prevention-source/obesity-definition/abdominal-obesity/.

ABOUT THE AUTHOR

Rovenia M. Brock, PhD, has been a leading nutrition coach for over two decades and a contributor to national media and news outlets—including National Public Radio (NPR), CNN, and HLN—as well as *The Meredith Vieira Show* and *The Dr. Oz Show*, where she has also served as a member of the show's medical advisory board for six of its seven seasons. She is the nutrition coach who helped more than a half-million Americans lose more than 5 million collective pounds in a single season. She is an award-winning nutritionist praised by *More* magazine and *ShopSmart* (the quick and easy guide from *Consumer Reports* magazine) for being one of the top five nutritionists in the country. She joins President Barack Obama, First Lady Michelle Obama, and Oprah Winfrey on *Ebony* magazine's Power 100 list of the 100 most influential African Americans in the United States (2010 and 2012). She is the author of *Dr. Ro's Ten Secrets to Livin' Healthy* and the e-book *You Healthy and Happy: Dr. Ro's Tips for Living an Inspired Life*. She is the nutrition director of Dr. Riggins MASC in Gadsden, Alabama, a practice she co-owns with her husband, Dr. Murray Riggins. Together, they live in Alabama with their beloved cocker spaniel, Simba, and their two labs, Bert and Ernie.

INDEX

Underscored references indicate tables or boxed text.

Roasted Potato Medley, 234
Sautéed Brussels Sprouts with
Carrots, 237
Sautéed Spinach, 189
Warm Steak Salad, 183
Dirty dozen, 59
Dried fruit, 141
Drinks
alcohol, 41, 83–84, 143, 158–59,
208
dandelion root tea, 257
fruit juice, 139, 141
fruits in ice cubes, 44
half your body weight in water,
43–44
mint-dandelion tea, 257
soda and sugary, cutting out,
44–46, 255–56

E

Eggs, 64–65
Electronics, avoiding in the bedroom,
42
Elrod, Debra, 254
Emotional eating. See also Cravings
bad feelings after, 23
celebrating with food, 22, 24–25
cravings journal for combating, 27
dealing with the feelings, 30–31
eating substitute foods, 28
failure of weight-loss plans due to,
20
gut check for, 29–30
learning from mistakes, 30
making better choices, 28–29
mindfulness about, 25–27
physical hunger vs. emotional
hunger, 20–22, 26, 258
self-medicating with food, 25
step-by-step plan for changing,
25–31
substituting activity for, 28–29
to cure pain, 22
Energy, boosting
exercise for, 7, 119
foods for, 6–7

lifestyle choices for, 7
mindful walking for, 133–34
thought strategies for, 7
Engineered cravings, 24
Evening shifts, special care for,
50–52
Everyday Vegetables. See also
Vegetables
list of, 56
in Phase 1, 79
in Phase 2, 140
in Phase 3, 205
Excuses for skipping breakfast,
39–40
Exercise
amount per day, xv, 117
amount per week, 249–50
bones and muscles strengthened
by, 119
calorie burning and, 117
checking with doctor before, 121
disease risk lowered by, 118
energy boosted by, 7, 119
as fun, 120–21
late in the day, avoiding, 41
longevity increased by, 120
most or all days of the week,
249–50
overview, xv
Phase 1 moves, 121–28
Phase 2 moves, 193–98
Phase 3 moves, 239–41
shift work and, 51
sleep aided by, 120
stress reduced by, 119
stretching after, 121
substituting for emotional eating,
29
warming up before, 121
weaving into daily activities, 139
weight loss boosted by, 118–19
weight loss maintained by, 117
Exercise moves
Advanced Level Pushups, 252
Advanced Plank Jacks, 252
Advanced Triceps Dips, 251
Alternating Lunges, 128
Alternating V-Ups, 196

reason for "15" in, xiii, 5
Self-Assessment Test, 9–10
simplicity designed into, 5–6
Fish and shellfish. *See also* Proteins
  eating the best you can afford,
    63–64
  grocery lists, Phase 1, <u>104</u>, <u>105</u>
  grocery lists, Phase 2, <u>162</u>, <u>163</u>
  grocery lists, Phase 3, <u>225</u>, <u>226</u>
  health benefits of, 62
  serving sizes, 61
  tilapia and farmed fish, 63, 66–67
Focus on life, rather than food,
    261–62
Food choices. *See also* Emotional
    eating
  decision points per day, 19
  eating substitute foods, 28
  emotional, 22
  emotions indicated by, 32–33
  energy-boosting, 6–7
Food diary
  recording cravings in, 27
  template, <u>48–49</u>
  using daily, 46–47
Food swaps, <u>248</u>, <u>254</u>, <u>263</u>
Fried foods, cravings for, 33
Fruit juice, <u>139</u>, 141
Fruits
  in the clean 15, 59
  in the dirty dozen, 59
  dried, 141
  fat-burning, 257
  grocery lists, Phase 1, <u>105</u>, <u>106</u>
  grocery lists, Phase 2, <u>163</u>,
    <u>164–65</u>
  grocery lists, Phase 3, <u>225–26</u>,
    <u>227</u>
  in ice cubes, 44
  not in Phase 1, 82–83
  as nutrient-dense, 140–41
  organic, 59
  Phase 2, 140–41
  Phase 3, 205
  serving sizes, 57
  sugar addiction and, <u>142</u>
  sugar cravings and, 82
  tips for choosing, 57–58

G

Genetics, diabetes and, 12
Ghrelin, 21
Gidley, Amy, <u>130</u>
Gluteal muscle exercise moves
  Alternating Lunges, 128
  Burpees, 123
  Jab-Cross Squat Combo, 198
  Jump Squats, 251
  Plank Jacks, 197
  Squats, 124–26
  Squats with Front Kicks, 241
  Sumo Squats, 193
Gluten-free (GF) diet, 70–71
Grains and breads
  avoiding refined grains, 69
  avoiding white grains, 70
  Ezekiel sprouted grain bread,
    69–70, 206
  gluten-free, 70–71
  health benefits of whole grains, 206
  noodles, 70
  not in Phase 1, 83
  not in Phase 2, 143
  Phase 3, 205–6, 208
  serving sizes, 68–69, 206, 208
  tips for choosing, 69–71
Grape-cubes for water, 44
Grocery lists
  pantry items for all phases, <u>103–4</u>
  Phase 1, <u>104–6</u>
  Phase 2, <u>162–65</u>
  Phase 3, <u>225–27</u>
  Success Strategy using, 47, 50
Guacamole, 68
Gut check for emotional eating, 29–30

H

Hardman, Brittany, <u>76</u>
Heart disease, 12–13
Heredity, diabetes and, 12
High Knees, 124
HIIT (high-intensity interval
    training)
  described, 122

HIIT *(cont.)*
    Workout #1, 125–26
    Workout #2, 195–97
    Workout #3, <u>242</u>
Hormones, physical hunger
    controlled by, 21
Hot foods, cravings for, 33
Hunger. *See also* Emotional eating
    cravings, 22–23
    eating breakfast and, 39
    hormones controlling, 21
    mindfulness about, 26–27
    not satisfied by fruit juice, 141
    as okay, 34
    physical vs. emotional, 20–22, 26,
      258
    reduced by weight loss, 34
    sleep's effect on, 41
    stress and, 131
    thirst confused with, 34

I

Iceberg lettuce, 55
Ice cubes, fruits in, 44
Insoluble fiber, 144
Intention, setting each day, 75

J

Jab-Cross, 239
Jab-Cross Squat Combo, 198
Jab-Hook Forward-Stance, 240
Journal. *See* Food diary
Jumping Jacks, 128, 196
Jump Squats, 251

K

Kickboxing moves
    Jab-Cross, 239
    Jab-Cross Squat Combo, 198
    Jab-Hook Forward-Stance,
      240
    Squats with Front Kicks, 241
    Squat with Alternating Side Kick,
      253

L

Leftovers, cooking extra for, <u>80</u>
Leptin, 21
Lettuce, trying different kinds of,
    55
Life, focus on, rather than food,
    261–62
Lifestyle choices, energy-boosting, 7
List, shopping. *See* Grocery lists
Longevity, exercise for increasing,
    120
Lower body exercise moves
    Alternating Lunges, 128
    Burpees, 123
    Jab-Cross Squat Combo, 198
    Jump Squats, 251
    Squats, 124–26
    Squats with Front Kicks, 241
    Squat with Alternating Side Kick,
      253
    Sumo Squats, 193
Lunch recipes
    Phase 1
      Lunchtime Turkey Rolls, 112
    Phase 2
      Black Bean Spaghetti with
        Tomatoes and Basil, 184
      Dr. Ro's Salad Dressing, 181
      Lunchtime Turkey Rolls, 112
      Mandarin Orange Vinaigrette,
        180
      Quick-n-Easy Tuna Lunch, 179
      Turkey and Herbed Cottage
        Cheese Tomato Wrap, 178
      Warm Steak Salad, 183
    Phase 3
      Dr. Ro's Salad Dressing, 181
      Green Tea–Pom Water Infusion,
        231
      Lunchtime Turkey Rolls, 112
      Mandarin Orange Vinaigrette,
        180
      Open-Faced Chicken Sandwich,
        236
      Open-Faced Shrimp Salad
        Sandwich, 235
      Quick-n-Easy Tuna Lunch,
        179

S

Stretching after exercise, 121
Substituting
    activity for emotional eating, 28–29
    for dairy foods, 60
    foods for cravings, 28
Success Stories
    Amy Gidley, _130_
    Amy Seymore, _248_
    Brittany Hardman, _76_
    Debra Elrod, _254_
    Drew Dale, _263_
    Jason Thomason, _203_
    Jawn Murray, _244_
    Johnjalene Woods, _139_
    Joyce Wilson, _199_
    Morgan Murphree, _142_
    Sherri Shepherd, _207_
    Susan Moore, _86_
Success Strategies, 37–52. _See also_
        F-15 Lifetime Success
        Strategies
    avoid eating within 3 hours of bed,
        41, 46
    cut out soda and sugary drinks,
        44–46
    drink half your body weight in
        water, 43–44
    eat early and often, 40
    eat snacks no larger than closed
        fist, 43
    eat within 1 hour of waking,
        37–40
    get 7 to 8 hours of sleep per night,
        40–43
    shop with a list, 47, 50
    take special care if you work
        nights, 50–52
    use a daily food diary, 46–47
Sugar
    in alcohol drinks, 84
    avoiding drinks with, 44–46,
        255–56
    avoiding foods with added, 81–82
    benefits of stopping, 82
    emotions and cravings for sweets,
        32
    fruits and sugar addiction, _142_
Sugar, blood, 11. _See also_ Diabetes

Sumo Squats, 193
Supplements, _85_
Support
    avoiding unsupportive people, 261
    community of like-minded people,
        260–61
    connecting to author on social
        media, 262, 264
    F-15 Facebook Group, 262, 264
    weight-loss support groups, 261
Swaps for foods, _248_, _254_, _263_
Sweets. _See_ Sugar

T

Tabata training
    described, 122
    Workout #1, 122–25
    Workout #2, 193–95
    Workout #3, 239–41
Test, Self-Assessment, 9–10
Thin thinking, 17–20. _See also_ F-15
        Mindset
    fat thinking vs., 18
    learning from thin friends, 18–19
    mindfulness for shifting to, 19
    money analogy for, 19–20
Thirst, hunger confused with, 34
Thomason, Jason, _203_
Thought strategies. _See_ F-15 Mindset
Tilapia and farmed fish, 63, 66–67
Timing and scheduling
    amount of exercise per day, 117
    amount of exercise per week,
        249–50
    avoiding eating within 3 hours of
        bed, 41, 46
    being the last one at the table to
        eat, 260
    buying produce in season, 54, 58
    eating early and often, 40
    eating within 1 hour of waking,
        37–40
    exercise late in the day, avoiding,
        41
    exercise most or all days of the
        week, 249–50